ON THE RAGGED EDGE OF MEDICINE

ON THE

Ragged Edge

OF

Medicine

Doctoring Among the Dispossessed

❧

PATRICIA KULLBERG

Oregon State University Press Corvallis

Library of Congress Cataloging-in-Publication Data

Names: Kullberg, Patricia, author.
Title: On the ragged edge of medicine : doctoring among the dispossessed
/ Patricia Kullberg.
Description: Corvallis : Oregon State University Press, 2017. | Includes
bibliographical references.
Identifiers: LCCN 2016049647 (print) | LCCN 2016050217
(ebook) | ISBN 9780870718854 (paperback : alk. paper) | ISBN
9780870718861 (ebook)
Subjects: | MESH: Kullberg, Patricia. | Vulnerable Populations | Delivery
of Health Care | Community Health Centers | Homeless Persons |
Socioeconomic Factors | Oregon | Personal Narratives
Classification: LCC RA418 (print) | LCC RA418 (ebook) | NLM WA 300
AO7 | DDC 362.1—dc23
LC record available at https://lccn.loc.gov/2016049647

First published in 2017 by Oregon State University Press
Printed in the United States of America

Oregon State University Press
121 The Valley Library
Corvallis OR 97331-4501
541-737-3166 • fax 541-737-3170
www.osupress.oregonstate.edu

AUTHOR'S NOTE

This book is written for my colleagues and coworkers at Burnside and Westside Health Centers, who were an endless source of wisdom and comfort to me during the decades of my practice. It is written in remembrance of all those folks, brave and imperfect, who entrusted themselves to our brave and imperfect care.

A special thanks to Barry Mattern for allowing me to tell his story and use his actual name in the narrative entitled "Imagine That." In all other cases names and identifying details have been changed to protect patient privacy.

I also wish to thank colleagues Diana (Anderson) Barnard, Catherine Ellison, Karen Hogue, Rich Houle, Pam Kelsay, David Pollack, Ollga Samarxhi, Cathy Spofford, and Mary Ann Ware for allowing me to include them in these stories. I wish I could thank our dearly beloved Izora Brown, but she is no longer with us.

I am grateful to Kathleen Concannon, Jonathan Eaton, Bob Henriques, Rachel Hoffman, and Linda Sladek for their gracious and helpful comments on earlier drafts of these narratives. I am especially indebted to my husband, Norm Diamond, and my son, Alex Diamond, not only for their careful and critical review of the manuscript, but also for enduring the years I devoted perhaps the best of myself to my colleagues and my patients.

My mother is a doctor at a homeless clinic in downtown Portland.
Because of the stress she experiences at work, she is sometimes edgy.

—Alex Diamond, age thirteen
From his essay "My Family"

CONTENTS

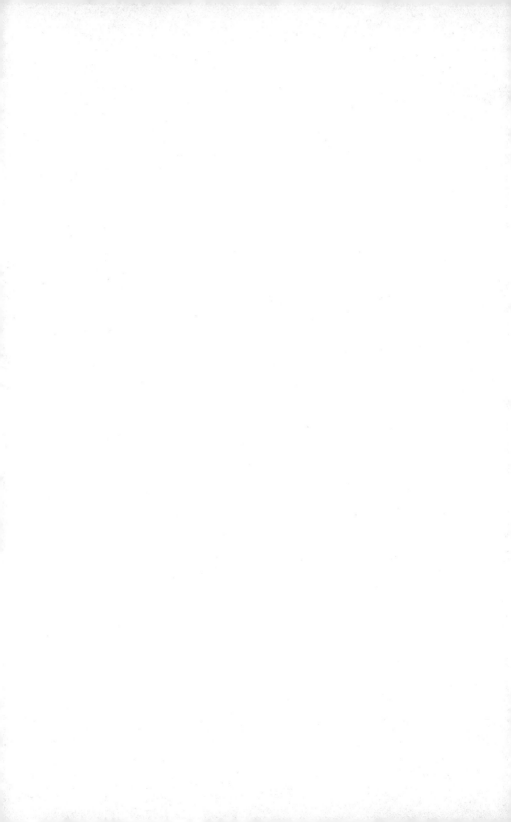

PREFACE

All too often a day at Burnside Health Center would begin with a mel-
ancholy tramp through the heart of Portland. I would leave my car in
the cool of early morning near the river that slices the city in two. The
parking lot spread out in the shadow of the Morrison Bridge, one of
ten bridges that spanned the river in those days. To exit on foot, I
passed under the downward slope of a curving off-ramp. Where it
came to ground, the ramp made a dank wedge of space, which often
smelled of piss and even in summer was spotted with oily puddles.
Sometimes, before a chain link fence was installed to keep people
out, I could make out blobs of sleeping bags at the farthest reach of
the space. Then I would look away, faintly embarrassed, as if I had
carelessly glanced into someone's bedroom.

From there it was a ten-block trek to the clinic. I would head away
from the river into downtown, merging with a bustle of suits, portfo-
lios, wingtips, and pumps, umbrellas in winter, shades in summer. I'd
pass cafés and more coffee shops than you'd think the market could
bear; a magic shop, a Western clothing store, and a business that ped-
dled vintage magazines; a glass and steel office building known as Big
Pink, because it was; and a couple of granite-faced edifices with the
names of Portland's forefathers engraved in the stone.

As I passed, I would scrutinize the overhangs, doorways, and parking structures for their merits as places to sleep. Could I squeeze in on
the dry side of that drip line? Could robbers, rapists, or thugs spot me
in that out-of-the-way corner? Would the north wind whistle around
into that recess? Would police or security roust me out of there in the

1

middle of the night? Weren't these the calculations that people living on the street would make when settling in for the night? The preoccupation was not a happy one, and whenever I caught myself refracting the streets through this particular lens, I'd force my mind elsewhere. I knew too many people sleeping out at night. They were my patients.

The best places to shelter, by my admittedly inexpert survey, were concentrated near the river and, surprisingly, on the skyscraper side of the north-south city divide, Burnside Street. Once I traversed the half-dozen blocks through the commercial core and crossed over Burnside to the north, I found no spots to spend a night beyond the shallow doorways. Here the skyline dropped on average a good ten stories; pea coats and T-shirts replaced the suits; sidewalks became littered with broken glass, smashed beer cans, and the soiled Styrofoam clamshells of fast-food takeout. Once in a while, in the gutter, even less savory items were discarded, like used needles or condoms. Instead of glass, steel, and granite, the structures were brick and wood, some of them dilapidated or boarded up, taverns with no windows, eateries with greasy ones, residential hotels, a shelter, a soup kitchen, and the remnants of a Chinatown in steep decline.

Near the end of the twentieth century Old Town, née the North End, where both the Chinese and African American communities got their start, was between two never-quite-complete attempts at revitalization. A jazz club, import megastore, and a couple of boutiques were left over from the last one. The next one would bring the Lan Su Chinese Garden, lofts converted to living space for upscale urbanites, and exclusion laws designed to keep habitual drug offenders out of the district.

Two blocks in I would reach Burnside Health Center, a storefront clinic on NW Davis, a street known to be the run of pimps, thieves, drunks, and dope peddlers. Next door stood the Butte Hotel, one of several SROs (single resident occupancy) in the area for lonely, down-on-their-luck folks, mostly men. The old hotel was infested with cockroaches, which streamed over into our space. We knew, because when the exterminators periodically arrived to spray the clinic, they told us that's where our roaches came from. Two blocks down was Sisters of the Road Café, where a person could get a meal in exchange for work. Burnside Projects (later Transition Projects) ran a shelter and cleanup center five blocks away.

My patients at Burnside (and later, at Westside Health Center, located in the commercial core) were poor and most of them sick to one degree or another. They were of every ethnicity and every imaginable blend. Lots of them slept under bridges, in parks, in their cars, or on their brother's sofa. Most lived with mental illness, addictions, or both. They included undocumented, disabled, and unemployed workers, sex workers, pensioners, panhandlers, and felons. Not a few of them labored in low-wage jobs. They were veterans of wars both legal and covert. Many of them didn't speak English; some of them couldn't read. A distressing number of them were on the streets because they were too cognitively disorganized to access the services to which they were entitled, like Social Security Disability.

The majority had suffered abuse of one sort or another, either as children, adults, or both, at the hands of family, institutions, and states. Some were refugees of war, coming from countries all over the world. Most were poorly educated, though among them was a doctor from Iran, a lawyer from Afghanistan, a nurse from Somalia. Also a musician, a journalist, a contractor, and a professor of physics, all native born and fallen on hard times or bad choices, usually a combination of the two. One said he'd traveled as a personal assistant to Red Skelton, and I believed him. Who would make that up? Most, however, had been poor their entire lives; not much ever trickled down to them. Economic boom or bust, it didn't matter; their poverty was a given.

They amazed me. They were funny, insightful, and caring in the midst of destitution. They were resilient and incredibly resourceful. Not for a minute did I think I could endure what they did. Far from perfect, they failed on many levels, and the consequences for their failures were severe. They suffered as well from my mistakes.

✿

I, myself, was a refugee of sorts when I came to Burnside, fleeing a suburban practice. The clinic there was spacious and light and included all the amenities of a modern medical institution. My coworkers were nice. My patients were lovely. Few were particularly sick. And I was terminally bored. I would catch myself watching the clock, the last thing I ever expected out of my advanced degrees in medicine and public health. I was itching to deploy my skills where they were really needed. I hankered for a practice that others would shun.

In 1988 I accepted the job of medical director for Multnomah County Health Department and became responsible for the quality of care delivered at what eventually swelled, over my two-decade tenure, to more than thirty primary care and public health clinical sites. For my part-time practice, I chose Burnside Health Center, located in the heart of Portland's skid row.

But it would be misleading to imply that I landed at Burnside out of a lust for intellectual stimulation and a desire to serve. I did. But that wasn't all.

✿

When we were growing up, my mother always had a "cleaning lady" who came weekly to help Mom maintain a modicum of hygiene and order in our large, three-story home in southwest Portland. Seven of us were a lot to clean up after. One time she hired an African American woman, a "Negro" she would have called her in 1953. Mom told the story that I, as a three-year-old, followed the woman around and pestered her incessantly about why her skin was so dark. The woman refused ever to come again. I have no recollection of the incident, but I do remember, as a schoolgirl, becoming entranced with a 1943 photo of my father standing next to a native of the jungle island where he'd been stationed as a flight surgeon for the Navy. The fellow had wrenched his shoulder out of its socket and Dad had maneuvered it back into place. In the shiny black and white snapshot my father towered over the other man, who was so dark I could barely make out his features. His hair was black and curly. He was clothed in what I took to be a short dress and no shoes. I had no idea men like that existed.

I was thoroughly white bred, an upper-middle-class WASP— white Anglo-Saxon Protestant. At college, during the tumult of the sixties, it became to me an identity that signified the opposite of cultural authenticity and moral authority. It bestowed advantages I had not earned. It had kept me apart from people of color and from those of the disadvantaged classes. It was sort of embarrassing, like something I had to make up for. I no longer felt quite at home in my own skin, among my own people, within the smug circles of privilege.

So it was that some sense of duty and middle-class guilt propelled me to Burnside, motives that can render the heart impure—patronizing and paternalistic. Clinging to the underside of that was the still more unworthy desire for adventure, to get a bit dirty without risk, to venture out where hardly anyone wanted to go. Medical slumming, you could call it. Suffering as spectacle. I see this now with clarity. Back then it was a vague discomfort that I suppressed. I had my self-image to protect.

The patients saved me. They took me at face value, as a doctor who was interested and wanted to help. They commanded my affection and respect. They taught me humility. They drew me in close enough that I could not be the voyeur standing outside and looking in, because I was no longer outside. I'd stepped inside, with them. Not that I ever did or ever could experience the depredations and humiliations of poverty that they suffered on a daily basis. But still, we became allies. We shared objectives. We cultivated the same institutional friends and battled the same bureaucratic foes. It was not, then, a tour of duty; it was no sacrifice to work there.

Over time I became more comfortable working with people whose life experiences were so utterly different from my own. The health department, through lectures and workshops, paid close attention to the issues of working across boundaries of culture, language, religion, ethnicity, sexual orientation, or gender identity and how to negotiate those differences with grace and respect. This is not to say that we always got it right. Still, there was an awareness, an openness and intentionality. What was mostly lost or ignored in those sometimes contentious discussions and presentations was class difference. We were lectured only on the culture of (white) poverty, which was interesting, though hardly adequate. Class was an uneasy topic, perhaps because we were all implicated.

I continued to struggle over the years with the problem of class privilege—inextricably intertwined, as it was, with white privilege— and the power dynamic it necessarily introduced into the exam room. I think it was because differences in language, culture, and experience were things to explore and celebrate. There was no justification, let alone joy to be had, in the unconscionable gap in wealth and privilege. It never escaped me that I went home to sleep in a bed and many of my patients went to sleep on the streets.

❧

These narratives are not about triumph and tragedy. They are about me and my patients, tussling with each other while struggling with the patient's physical and emotional distress, set in a context where conditions were pretty much stacked against the sufferer. It wasn't all that easy for me either. You won't find too many happy endings here. These are not my success stories. What interests us most, of course, is trouble. It is when we are in the grip of trouble, when things do not work out as planned, that we most often discover ourselves. I wrote these particular stories because what happened troubled me and the writing helped to clarify and illuminate. In some cases, it enabled me to forgive myself.

The stories are also reflections about the work of doctoring. The physical, psychological, and intellectual demands. The terrible uncertainties. The confines of the system we work in, with its twists and loops and blind allies, a system neither very rational nor functional, especially not in the outposts that serve the poor, out on the ragged edge of medicine.

I relied a lot on notes I kept about patients over the years. But I've reconstructed the dialogue out of my certainly sketchy memory. The timelines are approximate. The stories did not unfold exactly as presented here. Memory isn't like that. However, I have not strayed from the essential thrust of each story, the dynamics of what happened, and the impact on me and on my patient. It must be further noted that these are my versions of what happened; I cannot claim to know the fullness of the patient's experience. Still, the stories belong as much to the patients as they do to me. For an hour or for decades, we were parts of each other's lives.

FAST WATER

This time it was from a box of Corn Chex: a precise scissor cut around the green-colored word *Corn* offset above the big red letters of *Chex*. On the gray back of the cardboard cutout were printed the words *Indict the CIA*. Below that, as if I wouldn't know who'd left it for me, Jocelyn had scrawled her name.

🙖

Only one door opened into Burnside Health Center, not counting the one in the cellar, down a steep, poorly lit, and rickety set of wooden steps. The path through the cellar to that other door was one person wide through shoulder-height stacks of boxes. I have no idea what was in the boxes. They weren't our supplies, which we kept in an equally rickety loft overlooking the nurses' station. The cellar door, which was our nominal fire escape, was padlocked. The key hung helpfully from a nail next to the door. *I can't breathe! I can't see! Where's the fucking key!* We laughed about it. Most of what we laughed about was morbid.

Everyone entered the clinic—patients, staff, police, paramedics—directly into a tiny waiting room. Street dirt dimmed the only window that looked out onto the sidewalk. In front of the reception counter, thousands of soles had worn away the linoleum. Plastic chairs, sticky in summer, cold as the steel of a stethoscope in winter, lined the streaked and yellowing walls. On the wall hung a framed print of a wilderness scene—a rush of white water that tumbled over glistening rocks and looked to spill out into the room and wash everyone away.

When I arrived the day after the Corn Chex, several patients already occupied the waiting room. A disheveled old man with tangled white hair slept in the corner with his toothless mouth agape, a filthy knapsack and sleeping bag propped next to him. Likely he was the source of the slight smell of urine in the air. A couple of chairs away sat a much younger Latino man, mumbling under his breath. Across the room hunched a woman whose male companion sprawled in his chair, taking up too much space, ignoring his partner's distress. Not far from him perched a wraithlike figure with bright red lipstick, round spots of rouge on her cheeks, and straight black hair that plunged to her waist. She was applying crimson polish to her nails from a tiny vial she clutched between her knees.

Commanding the center of the room was a tall, stringy woman who paced in tight circles, peering at the others through narrowed eyes. The wild bush of her hair made her look that much more menacing, like some exotic creature puffed up before a predator. The other patients variously stared, cringed, or looked away.

She rushed up to me, swooping her hands through the air. "*Doctor Kull*berg! The good doctor is here and so am I may I join you in the inner recesses of your office where the battle is joined between *microbe* and *man*, between *white* coats and tweedle dee tweedle dum but she's not so dumb that Doctor Patsy . . ." Words flew out of her mouth like missiles. I motioned for her to follow me as she jabbered away. I cast a backward glance at our receptionist, Izora Brown, who gave me her thank-you smile. "Sit here," I told Jocelyn as I opened the door to the nearest exam room. "I'll be back."

Pam Kelsay, the lead nurse, rolled her eyes. Jocelyn was supposed to wait like everyone else. I was coddling her and undermining Pam's authority. I'd failed to hold the line.

Patients were known to hover at the opening into the hallway and ambush me as I exited a room. I never brushed them off, always let them take cuts, which interfered with Pam's careful control of clinic flow. Eventually, Pam moved me to the exam rooms way in the back and out of sight. It was the right move, and I was grateful.

Making excuses for people who are impaired, like allowing them to behave badly, can be a form of disrespect. A way to diminish them. It can, as well, sabotage their success in life. Meeting people where they were at, as Pam well understood, did not mean letting them walk all over you. It was one of my first lessons at Burnside. But I hadn't learned it yet.

I shrugged at Pam. "Sorry, she's bugging everyone out there."

"Are you going to talk to her?"

"Yes, I promise."

I dumped my coat, grabbed my stethoscope, and slipped into the room where Jocelyn was fidgeting in her chair.

"Doctor Kullberg medical woman, wonder doc, battler of the universe, medicine is exactly where *good* meets *evil*, or do I go too far? It's not really a *moral* battle is it Doc?"

"Evil and disease are often conflated," I started, but she talked right over me.

"Or is there *bias* and *prejudice* lurking in even the most scientific and *objective* medicine for *compliant* patients, they do whatever you say—"

"I would never claim—"

"What's eating you today Doctor Patsy, you're looking a little *tense*."

My shoulders were halfway to my ears. I let them drop.

"I hope I'm not the source of your discomfort. I'm here on a legitimate medical mission, my lithium level and no side effects you'll be happy to hear no dry mouth no tremor no diarrhea no confusion but *wait*! maybe that's saying too much whaddaya think Doc, am I confused?"

"Confu—"

"Now there's another whole story, quite a sordid one if you've got time to listen of course you do the drug companies thieves of the highest order—"

"Yes, I—"

"*Rob*ber barons! Modern day Rockefellers and Carnegies who themselves were instrumental, *more* than instrumental in fact . . ." And she was off again.

"Jocelyn! *Jocelyn!*"

She quieted for a second.

"I have to talk to you about your behavior in the clinic. The staff—"

"I'm in trouble again you know Doctor, I have to talk to *you* about something yes I do . . ."

I should have shut her up, moved on to the business of the visit. Instead, I sat back in my chair and crossed my legs. I was having fun.

"I *am* in trouble, my *case* manager, I'm a case all right, that pointy-headed narrow-minded little snit who's had all sympathy for the mentally ill bureaucratized right out of her and you know how they do that Doctor? They give them case loads that are so *huge* that even the most *self*-negating *term*inally empathic and *man*ic social worker couldn't begin to do justice to and then they make one eensy weensy mis*take* and they *throw* them—"

"I think you've got a point there, but—"

"She called me, that is *he* called me, my landlord said he'd talked to her and *they'd* decided, can you imagine that, without even consulting me, not that I would have any opinion on the subject only because it happens to be *me* that they're deciding about, but you know that happens all the time, I'm sure you do, that I would have to give up my hobby or give up, you have any hobbies? You look like the sort who would putter—"

"What's your hobby?"

Jocelyn leaned forward over the small table between us. "Collector! Collector of boxes of cereal soap sugar staples pills mothballs you name it a veritable history of US consumption going back decades in stacks neatly arranged paranoid they are about vermin and other disasters—"

Jocelyn interrupted herself to laugh raucously. "Phobias are a problem for more than just the lunatics—"

"What does your collection—"

"Vermin! It's all about vermin though I *do* maintain my nutritional status and my hydration that's important don't you think, especially for one who daily ingests the wonder drug lithium but *no* soda pop, bad stuff, ever hear about the struggle between Pepsi and Coke for worldwide dominion?"

She stopped to stare at me.

"So what are you going to do?" I asked.

"Oh I survive, the doctor shouldn't *hey*! You've got a new haircut, too short though isn't it?"

I frowned; she was right.

"*Hah!* The haircut *is* too short you know what they say about hair though Doc, it *grows*, take mine for example, I cut it myself." She winked. "Surprised they would let me own a pair of scissors? Well the truth is, I didn't tell them about the scissors, who are '*they*' anyway? ever contemplate *that* mystery of the universe?"

"Jocelyn, I need to have you—"

"You need to have me what? You and your—"

I held up a restraining hand. "You need to take a seat in the waiting room when you come for your appointments and please don't come early." I fired off words as fast as I could, trying to get it all out in the narrow gap between her monologs. "When you're talking with Izora—"

"*Doc*tor, *Doc*-tor I don't need a lecture, Pam's mad at me isn't she? Or is she mad at *you* for not controlling *me*? What an idea, that one person can control the other even in the context of mutual respect did I tell you about my time in Morocco, quite amazing . . ."

She was into another long rap, but at the breathless end she suddenly interjected, "I will behave myself if only for the privilege of coming to see the good doctor." Then she tilted back her head and laughed.

❧

Who would not be charmed? As it turned out, no one was but me. Jocelyn's wild pirouettes on the edge of madness were unnerving. Big-boned and sinewy, she projected a suppressed hostility that made everyone want to back away. She looked unhinged enough to do a lot of damage to anyone foolish enough to provoke her. But I always enjoyed her. Some patients reserved their best behavior for the doctor. I was the one who doled out the drugs, the excuses and certificates, the tests and referrals they thought they needed, the comfort and reassurance they did need. I was at once privileged and beleaguered. It was not unlike holding court. *Talk to your doctor today!*

With me, Jocelyn tried a little harder to keep her impulses in check. Or perhaps it was only because I gave her some space to let go the jumble of thoughts piled up in her head. The verbal release seemed to ease her tension. Her drive to talk was pathological. Pressured speech, we called it. I could never tell if she actually enjoyed talking or simply felt compelled.

A keen and critical intellect—albeit unencumbered by the usual social restraints—was evident in her flood of ideas. Jocelyn didn't give a rip whom she offended, including me. I was often inspired to dissect and explore her observations. But once a thought was out, for her, it was gone. To return to an idea, to savor it or argue it, was out of the question. Converting her monologue to a dialogue would have demanded repeated and forceful interruptions and an exhausting insistence on my right to respond. She was not a good listener.

Still she was, in many ways, an easy patient. She was never depressed; she didn't drink or use drugs. More than all this, she possessed a self-confidence and certainty of purpose, which many of my patients lacked. Or maybe it was simply manic energy. In any case, there was nothing pathetic about her. She was engaged with the world where others withdrew, and nobody messed with her on the street.

Jocelyn often brought cutouts for me from her boxes, scraps of colorful cardboard with handwritten messages on the back: *Reclaim your dignity! Work for world peace! The wars rage on, they just don't tell us!* The offerings would show up in my basket even when I hadn't seen her for weeks. I took it as a gesture of affection, and I appreciated her sense of outrage.

When Jocelyn first came to Burnside, she'd already burned her bridges at many of the local health and social service agencies: Burnside Projects, which provided a range of homeless services; Salvation Army, which had its own shelter and soup kitchen; Baloney Joes, another homeless service center; and Mental Health Services West, the downtown publicly funded mental health clinic. So we took her in. It was a point of pride. We took all those who were cast off by other systems for being too uncooperative, too unmanageable, or too violent. We'd give them another chance and sometimes it worked out. Sometimes not.

ɞ

"Jocelyn, I really appreciate your efforts these past couple of visits to sit quietly—"

"Do *not* patronize me Doc I understand the necessity of proper decorum within the hallowed halls of medicine where the sick and injured have gathered."

I listened as she waxed philosophical about the endeavor of medicine. All that wit and intellect exhausted in fruitless, frenetic activity. What a waste. I imagined her in command of herself, still quick and sharp, but capable of so much more. She'd be a riot to have an actual conversation with. If only I could have restored her mind to its natural brilliance.

She was already taking lithium, which had what we called a narrow therapeutic index, which meant that the difference between the blood level at which the drug became effective and the level at which it became toxic was slim. Even at proper dosing, it was a kidney killer. It was an effective but dangerous drug. Close monitoring was required. Years later it would be all but abandoned in favor of safer mood stabilizers.

"Jocelyn," I broke in. "Your lithium level is a bit low," I said, as if this were news. It was always low. "Wait!" I said as she opened her mouth. "I know you don't want to increase your dose. What about trying something different. There are some other medications that might work for you. They don't—"

Whack! She brought the flat of her hand down onto the small table between us. "*Work* for me, that's a clever turn of a phrase what exactly do you mean by *that*? Work to make me more com*pli*ant? work to undermine my collection? *Doc*tors, always wanting to get some chemical into my brain to control my thoughts, well they did that once *thor*azine made me into a fucking zombie." The tempo and pitch of her words accelerated.

"What do you like about the lithium?"

"I've *told* you the lithium helps me think, it frees my mind, it gives me clarity logic incisive thinking control of my faculties." She guffawed. "I see where you're going, you think you've got something better, *new* improved drugs for the lunatic, want to try a taste test Jocelyn? We've talked about this before, why do you *tor*ment me with these offers of bogus new and improved? Is there a little plastic prize at the bottom of this box? I thought we had an understanding, not true?" She glowered at me.

"Yes, we do have an understanding. Did you—"

"They kicked us all out you know everyone living there and some of those people really should not be living on the streets but I'll—"

"What are you talking about? Did you lose your apartment?"

"Progress! Development! A better Portland! The building will face the wrecking ball next week already you didn't hear? Smash, crash, balderdash!"

"Where are you staying then?"

"The waiting room of the ICU, no one has the heart to bother you, put a newspaper over my head, they think I'm some poor sap trying to sleep while my mother is dying, every night a different hospital it's not so bad there are worse places to sleep, shelters for example, now if you want to see *crazy* people just go to a shelter, but maybe Doctor Patsy is a little crazy herself?"

"Oh, I'm afraid so."

She scowled, then broke into wild laughter and I laughed with her.

🍎

For days, a late winter rain had poured down. The gray and feature-less sky descended so low that even in those rare moments between showers, the mist-thickened air clung to hair and clothing. People closed their umbrellas and resigned themselves to the wet. Then the temperature dropped, the clouds gathered into great white puffs and broke apart against a sapphire sky. A cold sun absorbed what mois-ture lingered in the air.

On the way back to my car I was drawn to the river's edge. The warm rain had precipitated an early snowmelt in the mountains, which drove silt-laden floodwaters into the river that coursed through the city to the sea. I stood at the wall overlooking the fast water. The river's normally indolent flow had quickened into a furi-ous pace, sweeping along branches snapped from streamside. They said it would subside by morning. Who were "they," anyway?

Jocelyn and I had shared a visit that afternoon. Like digging a pad-dle into the rush of the river at the wrong moment, I'd spun our little boat around and dumped us into the water.

"Hey Doc, whaddya think, I want to make a contribution, you know make the world a better place, I've not been *up* to it the past couple of years, but now a lithium-induced state of serenity grips me like in the old days, you must have been in college about then your-self, how old are you anyway or is that too *per*sonal a question?" She paused with a sly wink.

"I'm—"

"No matter Doc, no need to pretend, I did a little reading on bi-polar disorder, much better than the old label manic-depression, that word *manic* really does conjure up the image of lunacy doesn't it, do you think I'm a *lun*atic?"

"No, I don't."

She brushed over the disclaimer with a wave of her hand. "You wouldn't be the first, you can tell by the way they look at you, doctors are all pretty much alike, *very* edgy, they all want to get out of the room *fast*, even *you* lately I've noticed *you.*"

With a sharp intake of air she came to an abrupt halt. She cocked her head and stared at me. Her last words hung suspended in the silence between us.

I looked down and picked some lint off my sleeve. What had she noticed?

"So where should I volunteer?" She barked out a laugh. "Baloney Joe's? They could really use some help but maybe there're already too many lunatics working there how about the library they have an army of volunteers whaddaya think?"

I squinted at her and spoke without enthusiasm. "Sure."

"Except the lunatic might not work out very well, might drive everyone crazy unless she takes some of that modern-day thorazine, here look at this." She fished a cardboard cutout from her hip pocket, from a travel-size box of Colgate toothpaste. On the back she'd scrawled "Angela Davis has white teeth!"

"Bet they regretted *that* little mistake, letting her enter an institution of higher learning, amazing, gotta go Doc." She rose and strode out of the room.

❧

After that, her visits slowed down.

"You blew off your last appointment, Jocelyn. I was beginning to—"

"Wonder about me? Why would *you* want to do *that*? Why don't you wonder about where I'm going to sleep tonight you know I've worn out my welcome at the hospitals they are on to my game so what should I do?"

"There are always the shelters."

"Shelters!" she hooted. "The doctor wants me to go to a shelter!"

"I know they're not ideal."

"Not ideal! You have no—"

"Jocelyn, you're overdue for a lithium blood test."

She leaned way over the desk and scowled. "Lithium that's *all* you can think of, I'm more than a lithium-taking machine." She rose and stomped out.

Several days later she arrived in a frenzy. "I'm not taking any more of those pills don't help worth a shit just more *chem*istry better living through chemistry you believe that shit subliminal not so subliminal you know the studies but I *don't* have a chemical deficiency now do I Doc?"

She stood in the middle of the room, gesticulating wildly as I sat, wondering if I was stupid to let her get between me and the door.

"You don't have to take the lithium if you don't want to. But if you're going to take it—"

She started to speak.

I raised my voice. "Let me finish. If you want to stop the lithium, fine. Maybe you should stop it. But if not, I insist on blood—"

"She in*sists*, the doctor in*sists!*" She rocked back and forth from foot to foot, arms held tightly across her chest. "Always insisting, always telling me what to do always claiming that I'm a *dan*ger—"

"Danger? Did I say that?"

"Jocelyn *could* be dangerous because dangerous Jocelyn does not like doctors, not doctors who insist, not doctors who don't give a shit, I can't work with my stuff my objects of the universe, just another plot, you're so full of tricks I gotta have my *wits* about me YOU HAVEN'T DONE SHIT FOR ME WHAT DO YOU CARE!"

"I can't talk with you when you're yelling. I'm going to leave the room now."

I went to Pam and I bailed out. I told her that Jocelyn needed a new doctor. How could I treat a patient who had no confidence in me? Or one I found threatening?

Jocelyn was the first patient I ever fired. I discharged only two more patients over the course of my career, one for sending me a letter that explored in some detail his sexual desires for me, the other for harassing me on my home phone, an unlisted number she'd acquired through some sort of deception. With more experience, I would not have cut Jocelyn loose. Patients who were upset with me could always choose to see someone else. It was not my place to make that decision for them. Usually the bombastics were short-lived and they were not about me.

Not until years later did I realize I'd already bailed on Jocelyn months before I appealed to Pam. I'd given up on her. I'd lost patience. She'd become a chore, a hassle. I knew her so well, or thought I did, that I could no longer imagine her possibilities. She must have sensed what I hadn't even brought to my own consciousness and it trashed our relationship.

Once I stopped seeing Jocelyn, her behavior grew intolerable. She'd barge into the clinic demanding to see her new doctor. She'd charge into the back unescorted and thrust herself into Pam's face, towering over her with unmistakable threat. On her final unscheduled visit, Pam presented her with a letter she had at the ready, informing her that she was no longer welcome at the clinic. She never came again.

❧

Years after Jocelyn left Burnside Clinic and the clinic itself had closed, I ran into her in the lobby of the building where Westside Health Center was located, the new home of the Burnside practice.

"Dr. *Kull*berg! Here you are I trust you are well and still helping the long-suffering outcasts of society." She stood next to me in the elevator, grinning, words pouring out of her mouth. She was heavier, more haggard looking. She got off the elevator at Westside, still yakking at me over her shoulder. Clearly, she had a new doctor, one of my Westside colleagues. The letter of dismissal must not have made it to her chart. Or it was too deeply buried in the record. Or the staff had chosen to ignore it, to give her another chance. People did change.

We saw it all the time.

Within the month, Jocelyn was back in my practice.

✺

Living life in a constant state of hypomania can't be easy on the body. There is nothing *hypo* about hypomania; it simply designates a condition short of full mania, the pathological insomnia, frank psychosis, outrageous and dangerous behavior. By the time I started seeing Jocelyn again, she was into the press of old age. She'd grown gray and swollen. Her kidneys were failing.

I wasn't sure why she was suddenly mine again, but I was glad. It was her choice. She was giving me another chance. We never spoke about our earlier falling out. Someone had wisely taken her off lithium, which hadn't done her a load of good in any case and was too toxic for kidneys like hers. Maybe the lithium was to blame for her crappy renal function. She didn't seem to mind the fatigue and the swollen legs. She seemed happily oblivious to her precarious state of health. I was not.

She missed appointments, didn't take her medicines as prescribed. "Non-com*pli*ant!" she might have hooted at me years earlier, but she didn't talk like that anymore. Her blood tests would return with little red exclamation marks next to certain values related to her kidney function. Her potassium would climb to a hazardous level. I'd have my nurse track her down, adjust her meds, make a return appointment for a repeat lab. At that moment she'd disappear. For days or weeks. I'd picture her, facedown on the ratty rug of her apartment, her body rotting, her phone ringing off the hook.

Patients disappeared often enough, and often enough because they were dead. It made us anxious. Sometimes we sent a nurse to their home. Twice I went myself (I was not the only doc who did this, always on our own time) to find a patient whose well-being was at risk. We could also send out the police to do a welfare check, although this was not our favored option.

We once sent a nurse to Jocelyn's home. But most often Jocelyn would show up of her own accord, long after the time we expected her back, and maddeningly blithe.

I walked into the exam room one day, wearied but relieved to see her alive. She looked a mess. Her hair was greasy, her fingernails grimed. Her blouse was soiled with what looked like a week's worth of spilled food and gaped open between the buttons around her belly. She'd pulled her shoes off, the ones she couldn't tie anymore, because her feet were too puffed up with fluid. The skin of her feet and lower legs was mottled with dark pigment, the sign of long-standing edema. At one ankle, the skin had split from the pressure and oozed clear fluid.

"Jocelyn. Do you remember the nurse said you had to get another blood test to recheck your potassium?"

She looked at me intently, holding one stiff sock in her hand.

"I need to tell you, your potassium is no joke. If it gets too high, it can kill you. It can stop your heart."

She pointed at the split skin. "What do you think about that, Doc? Think it will heal, you know, with the foot all swollen like that, I've been trying to take care of it, but I thought I'd better come in and get your expert advice."

We sat without speaking for a moment.

"Did you bring your medicines?" I asked.

She dropped the sock and began rummaging around in the brown paper shopping bag she'd brought in. Out came a tattered pile of papers, a coffee-stained Styrofoam cup, a wad of red bandana, orange peels in a baggy. I was getting nervous. We discouraged the unpacking of patients' belongings in the exam rooms. It was a terrific way to import bedbugs and cockroaches. Jocelyn pulled out plastic pill vials, one by one, and set them on the steel tray I'd wheeled over for her.

"I've got something in here for you, Doc, I know you'll be interested, maybe it's in that pile"—she bent over to shuffle through the dog-eared papers on the floor—"I swear it's here, I put it in here this morning, just for you, I've been such a pain in the ass, it's not easy dealing with me, is it Doc, I know what I'm like, shit I know it's here…"

Pain in the ass? Was that a confession? An apology? A rare moment of insight? She didn't leave any space for me to respond, so I didn't, judging that none of the words I might have come up with would have made either of us feel any better.

I was wrong about that. Here's what I should have said.

You brought joy and laughter into my life. You made me feel appreciated. You shared parts of yourself with me that you didn't have to. You forgave me for losing faith in you. Or you forgot about it. In any case, you were more loyal than I was. We had fun together and I will never forget you.

A DELICATE BALANCE

She wore a dirty, red windbreaker, white stripe across the breast, on top of an olive green cardigan over a faded-to-no-color housedress that hung down past her knees and covered dark polyester pants, which dragged on the ground in little shreds off the heels of her filthy canvas sneakers. A button-up blouse with pale pink and blue blooms peeked out from beneath the housedress and under that, I could see the sagging neck of a ribbed, tangerine turtleneck. A striped knit cap was pulled down low over her brow. Among people living on the streets, the layers of clothing were common, usually because they provided warmth. On Joyce I suspected they represented layers of insulation against unknown threats. She was middle-aged, short and squat. She eyed me with suspicion and parried my questions with quick, guarded answers. So I quit asking. All she wanted was a refill of her Haldol, a jackhammer of an antipsychotic. Okay, I thought. It was our first visit. She was nervous. I would have plenty of time to make friends with her.

Joyce had been a regular at Burnside for years, cared for by a re-cently departed colleague. Better for her if she had been a patient at Mental Health Services West, which employed actual psychiatrists. We had lots of patients like Joyce, with chronic and severe mental ill-ness who would have been better served by specialists. Some of them were too functional to qualify for specialty services, where precious few dollars had to be spread over a large population—primary care for the poor was always better funded than mental health care. But lots of these folks refused to see a psychiatrist. They could not bear to think of themselves as mentally ill, certainly not so crazy that they had to go to a special clinic. For others, the prospect of going elsewhere was too logistically and psychologically daunting. A few were afraid if they went somewhere else, we wouldn't see them anymore. They trusted us. We were familiar. *Don't need to see no shrink, Doc. I got you.*

∙

Every month Joyce traipsed to the clinic for her Haldol and her Cogentin, the drug that tamped down the side effects of the Haldol. She never missed an appointment. She was never late. Always dressed in layer upon layer of worn, soiled, mismatched, ill-fitting clothing, menswear as well as women's, cheap garments, even when new. First thing in the visit, I would write her prescriptions, clear the task out of the way to relieve her anxiety about it. I made sure I never cornered her in the tiny exam room on my rolling stool. I kept my distance, though I missed the usual physicality of the doctor-patient relationship.

The laying on of hands was not only therapeutic for the patient, but satisfying for the practitioner. The warmth of physical contact cut both ways. There was also an aesthetic involved—in the textures of skin and hair or the colors and curves of flesh; the smooth glide of a joint through its range of motion or a tendon through its sheath; the rhythmic sounds of blood pulsing through the heart or air through the lungs; the astonishing perfection of the emergence of a nail at the end of a finger or the way the lower lid cupped the tears. Some pathological alterations were displeasing to the senses, but the majority were not.

In any case, Joyce didn't like to be touched. I refilled her drugs, offered various immunizations, recommended a pap smear, and whatall. She didn't want any of it.

In summer, once, she cut down to two cotton shirts, same polyester pants and knit cap. She sat with her hands cupping her knees. A couple of fans batted the hot air around the nurses' station and reception area. It was stuffy. She must have decided I was okay. We talked. I wanted to know where she lived.

At that time the homeless were concentrated downtown and along the inner east side of the river, under bridges and overpasses, on loading docks, in doorways or abandoned buildings. Farther out they camped in a friend's backyard or slept in their cars. Some of them camped in city parks, especially those with remote reaches, like Forest Park in the west hills or Oaks Bottom along the river, upstream from city center. As the population swelled through the 1990s, more people congregated in camps, one of them south of the Ross Island bridge, a location that had been occupied during the Depression by a squatters' camp, a Hooverville. Dignity Village, a modern tent city, was established downtown in 2000, dismaying many with its claim for the right to exist on public land. Right 2 Dream Too was yet another self-organized downtown camp for the homeless, established in 2011. Lots of people living on the streets avoided the shelters. Too crowded and noisy, disease-ridden, and rule-bound, too often patronized by the violent. Couples couldn't stay together in the shelters. No kids. No pets.

Joyce was sleeping "under a bridge."

"All by yourself or are you with someone?" I asked.

"My dog."

"I didn't know you had a dog. What kind?"

"Don't know. He's big." She thrust out her hand into the air to show me how big.

"What's his name?"

"Pooch."

I laughed a little. "That makes it easy. So, where's Pooch now?"

"They're keeping him, the other people that live there."

"So you have some friends." A small community of the tough and fragile and dispossessed. I imagined a tolerance, a fierce loyalty and protectiveness. Among them, what did it matter what had come before in someone's life? What mattered beyond today?

She shrugged. "They're keeping Pooch and my sleeping bag and stuff."

Her sole possessions. "Ever stay in the shelter?"

"They don't allow dogs."

I pursed my lips, musing. "They should have a shelter for people with dogs."

"Too many people."

"You mean in the shelter?"

"Shelter's too crowded."

I lifted her chart from my lap and parked it on the end of the exam table. She occupied the wooden chair next to the door, butt-worn and straight-backed, a no-nonsense chair, indestructible, like chairs for grade-school teachers. "Camping out's okay in the summer. I'm wondering about winter. Would it be better if we helped you get a place for the winter?"

"Don't know."

I made an offhand gesture. "You mind if I talk to our social worker? She might be able to help." Until then, we hadn't had a social worker. She was a blessing.

Joyce shrugged. "Room's a lot of trouble."

"Might be worth it."

She stared at me with slow-blinking eyes.

"I see you never miss a dose of your Haldol. It must do pretty well for you."

"Makes the voices go away."

I let those words nestle into the silence. "What are the voices like?"

"They're mean. They don't like me."

"What do they say?"

"They say I'm bad."

"What else?"

She moved her hands from her knees to her thighs, rested them there, pale plump hands on plump thighs, still as stone. "Don't know."

"What do you think about what they say?"

"They tell me to take a knife and cut my throat because I'm bad."

"Do you have a knife?"

"Pocketknife."

"Have you ever cut yourself with it?"

"I don't want to cut myself." Her face was blank, her tone flat.

I leaned back until I felt the sharp edge of the countertop dig into my spine. "How often do the voices bother you?"

"All the time."

"Every day?"

"Haldol makes them go away, but I can hear them anyway."

"What do you do when they say those bad things?"

Still that same expression on her face, like a woman alone, unobserved, preoccupied with what to do for supper—warm up the mac and cheese or send out for pizza. "I get in my sleeping bag and cover my ears."

"Does that help?"

"They go away."

"How often do you have to do that?"

"Pooch protects me."

"Pooch is a big help. So does that happen a lot, every day, once a week?"

"Don't know."

I sighed, immediately wished I hadn't. "You know, Joyce, I think we could get rid of the voices." I was sure we could.

She looked down at the floor.

"What about taking a higher dose of Haldol?"

"Tried that. It makes me stiff."

"If it makes you too stiff, we could also raise the dose of the Cogentin."

"It makes me too groggy."

"The Cogentin?"

"When I'm stiff I can't run if someone chases you."

"Chases you?"

"Bad guys trying to steal my stuff, trying to get me."

Abusers and rapists and thieves, trolling the streets for a victim, prowling for the special prize of a single, homeless woman. I felt sick. "Maybe we should work on getting you a room so you'd have a safe place away from guys like that."

No response.

"Well, how about trying something else? We have other medicines that can get rid of the voices like Haldol does, but they might not make you so stiff."

She looked up and spoke to a point in the air somewhere over my left shoulder. "Haldol works okay."

"Yes. The Haldol works for you, but you're also telling me it isn't quite enough, really, to get rid of those voices. We could even keep you on the Haldol and add a little bit of one of the other drugs, you know," I wrinkle my nose in a friendly fashion, "to try it out."

"It wouldn't work."

"I was just thinking we might be able to make it better for you."

"The voices are okay."

We never talked about changing her medicine again. It must have taken years for her to arrive at this delicate balance, this much Haldol and that much Cogentin, to manage the twin threats in her life: the voices and the predators. Who was I to fool with what she'd landed on?

✿

Once on a Saturday with Alex, my school-aged boy, in tow, I went to the clinic to retrieve critical information about a patient who'd been hospitalized. One corner away from the clinic, yelling erupted. Down the block a young man was screaming at no one in particular. He brandished a thin wood pole, making savage swipes through the air, jabbing it at invisible targets. He approached in a meandering fashion, at odds with the ferocity of his shrieks, scattering the onlookers. At a sprint, he would have been on us in three seconds flat.

Should we run? Toward the clinic? Could I unlock both the iron gate and the front door before he reached us? Did a woman and a boy look like people he wanted to hurt? If he attacked us, would anyone come to our aid? Could I protect Alex? Could I keep my own body between that man and my son? My heart was revved up and my stomach clenched.

What if I were Joyce? What if I had been alone with this man on the street? His only target, with no one else around, with no hope for rescue, and it was dark. He was young and strong and wild and I was small and old and weak. I was groggy and my legs felt thick and could not carry me with any speed. My brain was muddled, I couldn't think what to do, and voices were bawling at me. *You're bad! You should die! He's going to beat you to death with his stick and that's what you deserve!*

This was the closest I ever got to the terror and helplessness that Joyce must have experienced repeatedly. But my imaginings were only one scary episode removed from the abstract. I really did not, and could not, grasp what it was like for her. It was like having a baby. You think you know what it will be like, until you actually have one and realize the profound limits of your own imagination. Maybe Joyce got used to it, I would think. Maybe she was numb to her own vulnerability. Because what person could live like that? These were the ways I would comfort myself. For Joyce, I had no comfort.

That Saturday morning, the man stopped long enough for Alex and me to hurry, not run, around the corner, out of his sight, and safely gain the clinic.

❧

Early in the summer of 1996, Burnside Health Center closed. We had a budget shortfall. We always had budget shortfalls, but this one was bigger, the direct result of a new state arrangement to provide health insurance to more poor people. The Oregon Health Plan (a Medicaid program), brainchild of Oregon state senator (later a three-term governor), John Kitzhaber, MD, introduced the concept of feeding more people at the health-care table by thinning the soup. The entirety of health-care services were compiled into a list of diagnosis-treatment pairs, then ranked by the most critical and cost-effective to the least. Depending on how many dollars were available to fund Medicaid, a line was drawn across the list. Only those services above the line were covered. Obstetric services and nearly all cancer treatments were covered; diaper rash, most surgery for low back pain, and hay fever were not. Immunizations were covered; surgical repair for uncomplicated inguinal hernia was not, even if it were painful or restricted your ability to work. The approach made sense, but only if you gave up on the idea of comprehensive and universal health-care coverage.

The closure of Burnside Health Center was an unintended consequence of OHP, an irony born of the complicated funding scheme for federally funded clinics like ours. We laid off a nurse practitioner and moved operations five blocks south to merge with Westside, which was larger, cleaner, better outfitted, and better heated and air-conditioned. It occupied the fifth floor of an office building, a security guard at the main entrance.

We didn't like it. We preferred our tiny, stinky, leaky little nest over in Old Town. We knew how to layer against the heat and the chill. We could live with the cockroaches. We were used to the constant run of the toilet. We had Izora at the front desk, with her pyramid of frizzy hair and a smile sweeter than honey-pie, who called on her preacher-father's blend of love and discipline to rule over the waiting room. We had no clinic manager on site, only Pam, a blunt and hard-working lead nurse, who guarded the boundaries of those of us who got lax about that sort of thing. She only scolded us when we really needed it. When they shut us down, we exiled Burnsiders went into mourning.

A number of Burnside regulars, the patients that is, never made it to the new clinic. Joyce was among them. No message phone, no emergency contact, no case manager was in her chart. She was lost to us. Patients would disappear for months or years at a time, only to reappear with the same problems they'd always had. Their absences marked various events: incarceration, a failed move to another climate, a new job with health insurance, commitment to a mental institution, a relapse into drugs. Their return might signal a failure, a milestone of success, or a turning point. Regardless of circumstance, I always experienced a certain joy at reconnecting with those who came back. So many more disappeared and I never knew why. Their stories littered my mind like half-read novels.

§

Two years after her last visit to Burnside, on a bright and sunny March afternoon, Joyce showed up in my exam room at Westside. She wore the same knit cap, only a few layers of clothing, and a pair of sunglasses, which she never removed. She seemed happy to see me. I think I was more thrilled than she was. Yes, she laughed, she still had the same dog. She was living with "some girls" in an abandoned house. They had no heat, lights, or water.

When she found Burnside Clinic closed, she told me, she didn't know where to go, despite the sign posted on the door. She began visiting emergency rooms to get her refills. You couldn't have someone coming to the ER for a chronic condition, though. Clogged things up, a waste of time and money. They told her she couldn't come back. She should go to Dr. Kullberg, the doctor she couldn't find. When she exhausted the local supply of emergency rooms, she mounted the Greyhound to Washington, Idaho, or California. She only went just over the border to the closest emergency room, she reassured me. As if I were the anxious one. How incompetent and resourceful she was, all at once. Unless the story was a complete fabrication, always a possibility.

She was somehow transformed, not hugely, but she possessed an additional jigger of confidence. Maybe more nights on the bus or under the fluorescent glare of hospital waiting rooms and fewer nights out in the elements had relaxed her. Maybe the voices had trouble trailing her to all those exotic locales, across great rivers, deserts, and mountain passes in search of her Haldol.

Eventually she'd come to the attention of a local mental health crisis center. They took the time to examine the empty vials of Haldol and Cogentin that Joyce had packed around with her all that time. They had my name on them, and it must have been a simple task to arrange for her to see me.

It was for me a grand reunion. I never saw her again.

ON A BAD DAY

Her mother called me several days after they found Mindy. I'd never spoken with Mindy's mom before.

"I'm so sorry for your loss," I said.

"Mindy appreciated everything you did for her."

"I wish I could have done more."

"Her body was in terrible shape when they found her."

"That must have—"

"Four or five days she lay there. After that long, the rot gets into the flesh. The stench was terrible, of course, that's how they knew she was in there." She spoke as if she were advising me on the features of her favorite laundry soap.

"It was so bad I couldn't really tell it was her anymore, when they made me identify her." In a second, her voice shot from flat to furious.

"That doctor, who prescribed all those drugs? My daughter was a drunk! You don't give a bunch of drugs like that to a drunk. The idiot doctor should have known Mindy would take everything at once and kill herself. Giving a tranquilizer to a drunk! Who would do that?"

I opened my mouth as the line went dead. I was that idiot doctor.

§

Mindy always came to Burnside Health Center first thing in the morning, after the bars had closed and folks had dispersed from the nearby shelter (which kicked them out at the crack of dawn), but well before the fast food joints opened. Early in the morning, the ancient hotels of the neighborhood, converted years ago to residential buildings, were quiet and sleepy. Their elderly and disabled tenants had little reason to get up and out early.

She had only three blocks to walk to the clinic from her apartment. The line for the soup kitchen formed a number of blocks away. Likewise, the places where able-bodied men congregated to pick up day labor were a quarter mile off. People out looking for a fix hung out in the park several blocks distant from her route, or around the corner from the clinic in the opposite direction, in front of a dilapidated grocery, which someone later torched; it burned to the ground. Broadway, the main north-south drag through Portland's city center, bustled only a street away during the morning rush hour, but little of its foot traffic spilled over to the sidewalk along which Mindy made her way. All she was likely to encounter on her passage was an occasional fellow sleeping in a doorway or a stray pedestrian. Most days she could manage it. On a bad day, she stayed home.

She grew up the only child of a single mother. She never knew her father.

"What was your mother like?" I asked.

Mindy gave a tiny shake of her head, shrinking into her chair, the way she always did, as if she wished herself invisible. She looked small, a lightweight, and pale beneath a carpet of freckles, blonde hair in a coming-apart ponytail. She trembled like a woman on her way to the gallows. Her gaze was wide-eyed; she had a penetrating stare. It was unnerving, that look of hers, thrusting at me a demand I was not sure I could satisfy. It was as desperate a look as any I've seen.

"How did you guys get along?"

"She was okay." Her voice, like always, was quivery.

"Was she ever mean to you?"

Mindy shook her head again, more decisively.

"Did she ever abuse you in any kind of way?" Was I putting words into her mouth, this woman who had so few of her own?

Another head shake.

"How do you get along with her now?"

"She lets me stay with her sometimes." Mindy had been homeless off and on.

"That's good of her."

"When I was a kid, she made me eat everything on my plate. Even when I wasn't hungry."

"I see."

❧

"What have you got?" It was Dr. David Pollack, psychiatrist and medical director of the downtown mental health clinic, called Mental Health Services West during those years. I'd called him. He always took my calls.

"Twenty-nine-year-old female with agoraphobia. Her symptoms have been worsening over the past few years. At this point she's pretty much homebound. Spends days without leaving her apartment. She's never seen a shrink. Never been treated. No significant medical problems. She admits to a beer now and then with her live-in boyfriend. I imagine it's a lot more than that." Our rule-of-thumb was to double however much the patient admitted to drinking.

During those years, the arrangement of specialty mental health care (rearranged every half dozen years or so when things weren't working out, and they never did) had one overarching goal—to keep publicly funded patients, that is, poor people, out of the psych ward. Only those patients "at risk for hospitalization" were eligible for specialized mental health care.

Those at risk for hospitalization were the ones who wandered naked in traffic, refused to eat, tried to hang themselves, or swung their grandfather's sword at their landlord. Emergency room visits, no matter how frequent, did not count. The fellow locked in perpetual conflict with his neighbors over the poison gases they were pumping into his vents was not impaired enough for specialized help. Neither was the woman who took two hours to get out of her apartment, because first she had to turn off and unplug every light, the space heater, radio, TV, clock, hot plate, toaster, and refrigerator, then triple check each one to make sure it was dead. Mindy's suffering was, as well, too silent and too invisible.

David had great faith in the ability of docs like me to manage these patients and he was always willing to help. Years later he would become one of the region's greatest advocates for the co-location of mental health services within primary care, a model we eventually embraced. It made sense, especially given the burden of mental health disorders in our population. In my practice it was my single largest specialty referral.

With co-location, the patients were much less likely to get lost, literally and figuratively, on their way to a mental health provider, because that provider was three rooms away. We could use the "warm hand-off" by bringing a social worker or psychiatric nurse practitioner into the exam room during a primary care appointment. We could demonstrate to the apprehensive or reluctant that the mental health provider was really a pretty nice person. Warm hand-offs increased the likelihood the patient would show up for a later mental health appointment. Care coordination was vastly enhanced. How much easier it was to snag your colleague in the hall than call someone you might not know at some institution you'd never visited and where in the heck was their phone number anyway? How much easier it was to read the notes right in the same chart than have a patient sign a release, mail it off, and wait for the weeks it took to get the notes, if you got them at all.

I added a few more particulars about Mindy; David asked a few questions. "Put her on Elavil."

"Really?"

"Works great for anxiety disorders."

Amitriptyline (Elavil), and a couple of others in the same class, were the only antidepressants available to me at the time. (We had the MAO-inhibitors, but they were dangerous and rarely prescribed.) I'd never used Elavil for anything other than depression. Later on I'd use it for everything.

By the turn of the century the types and number of antidepressants had exploded and they were prescribed in ways that can only be described as promiscuous. The classes of antidepressants expanded to five or more, depending on how you counted. They were used for insomnia, anxiety, delusional and obsessive-compulsive disorders, and as adjunct treatment for bipolar, psychotic, and personality disorders. Some uses were what we called "off-label." Not illegal, because a doctor was licensed to prescribe anything she wanted for any kind of problem, based on her own good judgment. Off-label meant that the usage was not FDA-approved or recommended by the manufacturer, literally off the label. Elavil, for example, was used for headache, premenstrual syndrome, smoking cessation, eating disorders, neuralgia, and other forms of chronic pain.

The story was similar for other mental health drugs. Plus, they were used increasingly in combination. Mood stabilizers with tranquilizers. Antidepressants with antipsychotics and soporifics. Uppers with downers. Patients would sometimes come in on three or four, even five, psychoactive drugs at once, plus the drugs needed to manage the side effects of the psych drugs.

But when I met Mindy, it was the late 1980s. We had many fewer options. Nearly every mental health road led to Elavil.

❧

She'd taped her glasses back together at the bridge. Beneath the lens, the left eye was swollen, not too bad. Purple and green had spread down onto her cheek. It looked several days old.

"Your glasses are broken," I said.

"Uh huh."

"Let me see that eye."

She pulled the glasses off for me to examine her black eye.

"It's healing up fine." I sat back down on my stool, crossed my legs, clasped my hands around my knee, my thoughtful and unhurried pose. "How'd that happen?"

"We were drinking."

"Did Ted do that?" Ted was the live-in. I wasn't sure if he paid the rent, or she paid with her disability check and he sponged off of her, not an uncommon arrangement.

"He was drunk."

"Has he hit you before?"

"He gets drunk sometimes."

"How often?"

"Not very often, just the weekends. Sometimes."

"And then he gets mean?"

She looked away.

"Are you guys drinking together a lot?"

"Sometimes."

"You know, Mindy, it's not okay for Ted to hit you."

"It only happens when he's drunk. He just gets stressed out sometimes. It's really hard for him."

"It's still not okay."

"It's my fault."

"Your fault?"

"I'm . . . too difficult."

"How are you difficult?"

"You know how I am."

"It does not matter how difficult you think you are. It's still not right."

She searched into my eyes with that wide-eyed look. "He always feels bad after he hits me."

"If you're afraid to leave him, I can help you with that."

"I don't want to leave him."

§

"She took the Elavil every night for six weeks," I told David over the phone.

"What dose?"

"One-fifty. She's not very big. I feel like I'm pushing my luck." Elavil was toxic at high doses, to the heart, the liver, the brain.

"Side effects?"

"Not especially."

"You could go to two hundred."

"But I'm worried she's got a lot of alcohol on board. She says it keeps her from having nightmares." The booze probably worked better than the Elavil to calm her down and was certainly easier to get. But it added to the risk of toxicity.

"You could get a blood level."

"You know, David, I really don't think we should be trying to manage her here."

There was no point in saying it. Aside from the fact that she was not impaired enough to meet their criteria, the mental health clinic would not take Mindy until she sobered up. But the alcohol and drug treatment agencies would not admit her until her psychiatric symptoms were controlled. That catch-22 landed a lot of patients in our lap. Substance abuse was nearly three times more common in persons with mental health disorders. A third of all mentally ill persons struggled with addiction and the rates were even higher among those who cycled in and out of prison, drug treatment centers, and specialty mental health clinics, like so many of our patients.[1] Alcohol and drugs offered temporary relief of symptoms. Patients used them to self-treat.

But we were ill equipped to manage this complex of problems. Back then we had no social worker, no psychiatrist or psychiatric nurse practitioner, no case manager, no alcohol and drug counselor. Both sides of the behavioral health world would eventually embrace the idea of dual diagnosis and the necessity of treating mental illness and substance abuse simultaneously. But during the time Mindy was my patient, we were on our own.

"I wouldn't be doing much more than what you're doing," David said, trying to shore me up. It wasn't like he had good choices. "I'd put her on Prozac."

"I've never used it."

Fluoxetine (Prozac) was the miraculous new option for treatment of depression with a novel effect on brain chemistry. It was the first selective serotonin reuptake inhibitor (SSRI) to be released. It was safer in those who drank. The lackluster performance of the SSRIs in all but the most severely depressed would not be exposed until after the turn of the century.[2]

My habit was to avoid new drugs until they'd been out for several years, to flush out any unexpected adverse effects. Let someone else experiment on their patients. Besides, new drugs were always pricey and we were poor. Because the majority of our patients had no health insurance, we dispensed drugs for a nominal fee that was usually waived. What was the point in taking care of people if they couldn't get the medicine they needed? However, our budget for pharmaceuticals was small. We had a list of drugs we could prescribe. Prozac was not on it.

But doing nothing for Mindy was not a great option. I put in for an exception, a therapeutic trial of Prozac.

❧

Several days after starting Prozac, Mindy showed up at the clinic. She stumbled into the exam room, lurched against the table, and spun around. "I can't stand it anymore!" she wailed. "You've got to help me." Her speech was slurred. She smelled like booze.

I'd always thought of her as a small woman. Seeing her now, swaying on her feet, I realized that she was both taller and heavier than I was. I sat her down and made some calming noises.

"I can't eat, I can't sleep. What's happening to me?!"

"When did all this start?"

"Ted told me he'd kick me out if I didn't settle down!"

"Did something happen between the two of you?"

"He's says I'm crazy."

"Is your mom around?"

"I don't know. I don't know where she is. There's nothing left to do but kill myself!"

Finally, I left her there, intending to beg someone to admit her. I'd never seen her like this. Her anxiety had never been more than a whisper, a tremble, a wide-eyed stare. She'd never made any kind of suicidal gesture, had never even talked of killing herself before. But I couldn't be so sure. Something was terribly awry.

I didn't even reach the phone before a crash reverberated through the clinic. I raced back to the exam room.

Mindy had knocked the otoscope, ophthalmoscope, and blood pressure cuff off the wall. She'd swept all the supplies off the counter: tissues, a box of gloves, push dispenser of rubbing alcohol, steel canisters of cotton swabs and gauze pads, small boxes of slides and cover slips. Then she'd broken a glass slide in two and dragged the jagged edge across her wrist. A thin ribbon of blood was oozing into view. When she saw me, she broke down into sobs. I pried her fingers loose from the broken glass and wrapped gauze around her wrist.

She offered no resistance, but the two burly cops who came to haul her away slapped her into handcuffs. It was disturbing.

Later that year reports surfaced about "Prozac madness."[3] The media sensationalized the stories. Still, in susceptible patients, Prozac could induce extreme agitation, even suicide. I never again prescribed it for a patient with anxiety.

§

"You look good, Mindy."

She wasn't shaking. She even had a smile for me. She'd spent four days in the hospital, long enough to wash out the Prozac, start her on something new, and determine that she didn't need a psychiatrist. That suicidal gesture of hers was pure Prozac. Her primary care doctor could manage her just fine. I'd thought for sure she'd earned her right to specialty care.

"The new medicine is helping me a lot."

The psychiatrist had prescribed alprazolam (Ativan), a close cousin to diazepam (Valium). He gave her enough to last until she saw me.

"I can sleep now, and guess what, Dr. Kullberg. I'm not drinking. I quit."

"I'm really happy to hear that."

"The psychiatrist said it would be dangerous with the new medicine."

"I agree."

She looked down into her lap and smoothed her pants over her knees. "Ted's gone."

"You mean for good?"

She nodded without looking up. "He left me."

"Before or after you went into the hospital?"

"While I was gone. He moved out of town."

I touched her knee. "I'm sorry. I'm sure that's not what you wanted."

She stayed silent.

"A break-up is never easy. But maybe it's for the better."

She looked up and smiled. "I think you're right."

I could tell that it pleased her to please me. It might have been what she was most happy about that day. Isolated and dependent, she had little opportunity to enjoy the pleasures of doing something for someone else. Getting better would make me happy and that would help strengthen her resolve. Some patients worked harder to please me than to please themselves, and I exploited the impulse ruthlessly. Like a parent would, and, like a parent, I hoped and assumed they would eventually come to do for themselves. It was always better when they worked to their own satisfaction.

I pulled out my prescription pad and stopped a second, my pen hovering over the paper. I never would have started Mindy on a drug like Ativan. It was addicting. It would do nothing for her in the long run. It was the last thing I wanted to throw into the pot with alcohol. Two weeks sober was not all that reassuring. But the psychiatrist had judged it the right therapy for Mindy at this point in time and sitting with her that morning, it seemed he was correct. I wrote the prescription, another two-week supply, and told her I'd see her then. Give her a period of relief, I thought. Get her over the alcohol withdrawal. I could wean her off the Ativan later.

I thought a lot about that visit afterwards. I should have done this. I should have done that. I should have known. I should have expected. I thought about Ted, as well, or rather, the abrupt way he abandoned Mindy. He was the only friend she had. One thing I'd learned early in my career: a patient could endure most any kind of suffering, if she were not alone.

❦

Several days later Izora buzzed me from the front desk. The medical examiner was on the line. I hated those calls; they meant someone had died. It was almost always someone I didn't expect. It was always shocking. The name would penetrate my ear and a hot chill would wash over me.

Mindy had lain in her apartment for some days before the police, alerted by her mother, broke in. Empty pill bottles were scattered about. Toxicology tests revealed that she had died of a combined overdose of (leftover) Elavil, Ativan, and alcohol. She'd taken every pill she had on hand. She killed herself only a few days after she'd seen me and one week shy of her thirtieth birthday. No memorial was held. Who, except her mother and me, would have gone?

IMAGINE THAT

Antisocial Personality (aka: jerk, asshole, butthead): egocentric, unethical, exploitive, deceitful, remorseless, coercive, manipulative, callous, hostile, irresponsible, impulsive, criminal

He was unsteady on his feet, from the booze, the beating, or both. Someone had stuck him in a wheelchair and rolled him into the exam room. One eye was swollen shut, his lip was split, and a gash over his left brow was stitched closed. His shirt was splattered with blood. He was drinking again; when sober, he didn't get into fights. I wasn't surprised. Not even dismayed. I was annoyed. He was making extra work for me on a busy day. Everyone else had to wait while I waited on him.

"So, what happened?"

Barry's voice was graveled. "There were these two little shits, came into Dugo's lookin' for some sucker to sell their junk to." Dugo's was a dive bar on Burnside. "I chased them out. I don't like those bastards coming down here."

Barry had standards.

"After I left, they jumped me from behind, little shit cowards, had me down before I knew what hit me. I think they had a two by four or something, hell, I don't know."

They'd beaten him unconscious and left him crumpled on the sidewalk. Paramedics had scraped him off the concrete and run him up to the hospital. Still tanked and furious, he'd told the doctor a thing or two about the crappy care he was getting.

"Shit, they stick you in these little cotton deals," he explained to me, "and I'm freezing and my head hurts like crazy and they don't give nothing for pain, they say 'cause I'm drunk. Figure I can wait forever because I'm an old drunk, sonsabitches. What the hell they care."

He'd staggered out before the eye doctor arrived on the scene. The misery of the bus ride from the ER to downtown, all that rolling and jolting when his head was pounding and his stomach ready to heave, effected a change of heart. He came straight to me.

But I couldn't pry his eyelid open to examine the globe beneath. He needed someone who knew what they were doing. Like an ophthalmologist. I was nervous about the eye. He wasn't.

"You see, Doc, I gotta sober up. You know how sick I get coming off a drunk. Last time I had a seizure. Man, that was bad. You remember. I'm too sick to go to Hooper. I gotta go to the hospital." He hung his head, all woe-is-me.

Hooper was the local sobering station. If Barry had to sober up in the hospital, it wasn't because the beds at Hooper were crappy, the food was worse, they denied you all privacy, and they bugged you constantly about your drinking and what was your plan for staying sober, a playbook Barry knew front to back and upside down. It wasn't because he was so plastered they might make him spend the night in the tank on a concrete floor, pissing and puking himself and where was the dignity in that? He knew I'd have no sympathy for any of this. He had to sober up in the hospital because he was too sick, anybody could see that, and, of course, Dr. Kullberg, his personal physician, would understand.

The hospitals would not admit a person with uncomplicated alcohol withdrawal, even guys prone to seize. They loved Hooper. All those drunks and junkies, most of them destitute—the hospitals did not want them soiling their beds. But the head and eye injury did change things. Hooper wouldn't take Barry. I set up the admission for him, feeling a bit like I'd been had.

"Barry," I said as they rolled him out, "don't be a jerk. It doesn't help when they're mad at you."

He lasted two days at the hospital, walking out AMA (against medical advice) late one night after getting into a shouting match with another patient, whom, he later told me, was a buddy of his.

§

Many, many years earlier, when I'd known Barry Mattern only a year, I had occasion to request his old medical records. This was at Burnside, before I'd convinced enough people it was a waste of resources for a doctor to do clerical work. I pulled out a request form, in triplicate, penned in his name, and looked up. "You ever go by any other name?"

"Butthead," he said. His smile was a contest between cocky and chagrined.

§

Barry couldn't remember what his mom looked like. She'd been locked up before he turned four and he was never allowed to visit. She had schizophrenia or manic-depressive disorder, or something, what did he know? It was right after World War II. Maybe she was rebellious. Women who got tired of their dust mops and Betty Crocker cookbooks sometimes got stashed away against their will. His father was stern, close-mouthed, and quick to the fist, boot, or belt, a military lifer whose assignments took him to far-flung places, and most of the time he didn't want to drag his brat along. For a few years, Barry lived with a grandmother he remembered as kind.

His dad eventually remarried and left Barry in the care of his new stepmother. When his dad whacked him, Barry knew why. He was predictable, and Barry figured he probably deserved every lick he got. But the stepmother? She beat him for any and all reasons and for no reason at all. By his early teens, he'd gone wild and a lone parent was no match for him. He'd already begun to drink, which only seemed natural. His dad and various grandparents, aunts, and uncles were all a bunch of drunks.

At sixteen he landed in St. Gabriel's Hall, a mid-century version of a lockup for incorrigible teens. A fist in the face was sometimes employed to keep the kids in line. It was a more respectful gesture, Barry felt, than the most common discipline: a bendo board (short for *bend over*), with holes drilled into it to reduce air resistance, administered whenever possible as the boy emerged from the shower with bare, wet buttocks.

They released him after eighteen months, straight into the army. It was the sixties and Barry was itching to go to Vietnam. But as the only surviving son of his father, the military brass refused to send him into combat. Furious about the lost opportunity to kick some butt, Barry served out his time in Germany and achieved an honorable discharge. Within several years he'd married and divorced twice. The second union produced a son. During his wife's pregnancy, he checked into a hospital to sober up. The alcohol was doing his marriage no favors. But by the time he got out, the wife had split with his baby. He never saw either of them again. In the wake of this loss, he tried to kill himself.

He held a series of jobs, but never latched onto any career. His life revolved around drinking. In the mid 1980s he killed a man with his car; he was drunk at the wheel. They threw him into prison. During his incarceration, he ran a marijuana import business. He calculated he made about forty grand during his six years of lockup. It was a little hard to believe.

He once wrote and posted a manifesto about the crappy prison conditions, the food, hygiene, being forced to buy his own clothes. For that they threw him into the hole for a couple of weeks, then sent him from medium to maximum, where no kind of writing materials were allowed.

I met him in 1990, not long after his release.

※

At that first visit, Barry was a sorry looking character. Tall, big-boned, and gaunt, he walked with feet spaced wide apart. Decades of drink had poisoned his nervous system and wrecked his sense of balance. A shock of white hair framed his deeply lined face. He managed to look both tough and pitiful.

"I'm a big drinker," he told me. "No point in pretending otherwise." He was a heavy smoker, too. What alcoholic wasn't?

He felt terrible. He complained of stomach pain, chest pain, vomiting, diarrhea, weight loss, shortness of breath, and a racking cough. During the exam he was struck by a fit of coughing and vomited.

Most of his problems I could write off to the booze and fags. But he looked pretty sick, even for a big drinker.

※

Tuberculosis (aka: consumption, white plague, Victorian novel disease): fastidious, opportunistic, sly, sinister, slow, mysterious, mutable, resistant, relentless, deadly

Barry was a classic modern-day American consumptive, a resident of the downtown streets and dives, whose immune system was shot by the depredations of alcohol, tobacco, and poverty. TB thrived where people were weakened by chronic disease, malnutrition, and substance abuse. It spread where living conditions were unsanitary and crowded. The only other reservoirs of infection in the United States were among immigrants from developing nations, who imported it from their countries of origin, and among those with HIV disease. Many physicians would never see a single case of TB in their entire careers. Barry was my third in two years.

Two large areas of tuberculous consolidation had been smoldering, one in each of his lungs, for months or perhaps years. Once the bacilli gained a foothold, they settled in for the duration. They had the nasty habit of sequestering themselves in out-of-the-way places, surrounded by layers of scar tissue laid down by an unsuspecting host, biding their time until the host's defenses were weakened by some debilitating condition. They could wait for years. They could infect just about anyplace in the body—bone, spleen, kidney—but they loved the oxygen-rich environment of the lung. Before antibiotics, the more drastic treatments for pulmonary TB included squashing the oxygen out of the lung with sandbags or injecting air into the chest to collapse the lung for the same effect. Sometimes surgeons cut out the infected mass, but the surgical approach rarely worked. Bugs were always left behind.

Now we flooded the bacilli with drugs, four of them at a time, for six months, minimum. If you pussyfooted around with one or two drugs, the bugs mutated into resistant forms. Many of the anti-TB drugs were hard on the liver.

No one wanted TB skulking through the streets, shelters, and cheap residential hotels of downtown Portland. It wasn't all that contagious, but in the cramped quarters of a shelter it could be murder. I called in the TB controllers. Another employee of the health department, Dr. MaryAnn Ware, affectionately known as MAW, took over.

§

Barry, appalled by the idea of being eaten alive, stops drinking and takes his medicine, every day, in front of a nurse in the TB clinic. He gains weight, stops coughing, feels great. The cavities in his lung shrink down to nothing. But after two months, he can't stand it. He falls off the wagon. The TB outreach worker has to track him down at Dugo's, drinking at the bar, to deliver his medicines. His unhappy liver swells up.

MAW, not interested in killing his liver, stops all drugs.

Barry, after a few weeks of alcoholic misery, climbs on the wagon again and restarts his medicines. But his liver has had it.

MAW tries this and that combination of drugs; she can't get away with anything. His liver has a chip on its shoulder. Anything he takes, it flares up. He starts drinking again. She orders more X-rays. She sees no sign of infection, but that's a false consolation. The bugs are there; we know they are, but they might throw up the white flag. Uncertainties prevail. But MAW is a good doctor. She knows when to quit. Before she does . . .

Barry bursts into my clinic and demands a prescription for pancreatic enzymes. He's losing weight, pukes every morning, his stools are watery, and he feels like shit. The enzymes fixed up a buddy of his. They'll fix him up, too.

I tell him he smells like alcohol and I'm not giving him any enzymes.

Barry starts yelling. *You don't want to help me! You're just like all the others.* He slams his way out of the clinic.

Two days later MAW forwards me a voicemail from Barry, directed at the two of us. It is profane and derogatory. We're fired.

We're amused. We don't take it personally. The outcome of the epic battle between Barry and his consumption is yet to be written.

𝕊

Five months later Barry showed up again. I was not surprised. It was not the first time a patient had fired and re-hired me. He'd been drinking pretty steadily and had the same litany of complaints. Not a word was exchanged about our last meeting or the phone message. But once he came back to the clinic, he was unfailingly polite and respectful, to me and the staff. That's not exactly true. He once called me up, impersonating a doctor to get beyond the front desk, to extract information from me he apparently thought I would refuse to give him. The ruse quickly unraveled. On the next visit he apologized profusely, embarrassed by his own behavior.

I couldn't do much for the slow, self-inflicted alcohol and nicotine poisoning except point out that I couldn't do much. Plus, I reminded him, he was inviting TB back into his life. Then what? He'd succumb to the bugs or the drugs, one of the two. He didn't dispute it. Periodically, I ordered a chest X-ray. Aside from his emphysema, they were always clear. After a few years, MAW said there was no point, unless he had symptoms.

During one of his dry spells, I suggested a trial of an antidepressant. I couldn't reliably diagnose depression when he was drinking. Alcohol itself was depressing, and it took a few months to get out from under its effect. He was rarely sober that long. The couple of times he was, he seemed pretty upbeat. Pinning a diagnosis of depression on him was a stretch. But it couldn't hurt to try. My idea was that it might keep him off the sauce.

After a few weeks, he quit the drug. "It got in the way of my drinking," he explained.

❧

One holiday season, Barry was admitted to the hospital. He was bleeding from his gut, and the salts in his blood were depleted to a dangerous level. It was the sickest he'd ever been from drink.

After that, his days of sobriety began to outnumber his days of intoxication. His periods of intense drinking shortened. Even when sober, he used to hang out in bars drinking soda pop. Now he avoided the drinking establishments, quit the life altogether. But without the alcohol to structure his days, he didn't know what to do with himself, so he enrolled in school to study computer science. Imagine that, after thirty-five years of drinking. It was challenging, but he stuck with it.

❧

"A psychiatrist in prison diagnosed me with antisocial personality," Barry told me once. "What do you think?"

Yeah, probably right. I hadn't thought about it, didn't see the point in confirming that particular diagnosis. It wouldn't change a thing. Or . . . maybe it would, for the worse. If you know you're a bastard, you'll act like one. We all have the urge to live up to who we are.

"I don't know, Barry. You're always nice and respectful to me." Which was true.

I could see he wasn't used to being told he was a nice person.

§

A disease is something you have. It is alien, separate from you. It strikes, assaults, invades, afflicts, always from the outside. Even those with mental illness usually retain a sense of themselves apart from the craziness they suffer. As symptoms wax and wane, they feel less or more like themselves. They know, or can imagine, who they are, absent their particular disorder.

A personality disorder crosses over the line between self and not-self. It is not something you have; it's who you are. It's an enduring set of traits at the core of your being—for example, being habitually paranoid, narcissistic, eccentric, or hysterical. Barry didn't *have* buttheadedness. As he was the first to tell me, he was a butthead. What does it mean, then, to conceive of a person, in his essence, as pathological? What are the implications for therapy? Can you even call it therapy when the object is to fundamentally alter the personality?

Personality disorders don't respond well, if at all, to drug therapy or to any kind of psychotherapy. We'd try, with various behavioral interventions we jokingly called "re-parenting." In recognition of their intractable nature, personality disorders were "below the line" on Oregon's famous list of diagnosis and treatment pairs. Medicaid in Oregon would not pay for any kind of treatment for personality disorders.

§

During a break from school, Barry took to drink again, selling his treasured computer to liberate cash for the booze. The binge lasted only a week, but it was long enough to land him in the ER at the Veteran's Hospital, where they did a routine chest X-ray. He had a mass in the left upper lobe of his lung. The doctor ordered a CT scan of his chest. It had the characteristics of cancer. In addition to the mass, he had several enlarged lymph nodes around the great vessels of his heart, presumably pregnant with malignancy. Not unexpected in a lifelong smoker.

The docs at the VA knew Barry had a history of TB. MAW and I reviewed his case. We let them proceed.

The surgeon gave Barry the option of having a transbronchial biopsy of the mass or having his chest cut open to remove the lump in its entirety. The former meant snaking a tube down his windpipe and guiding a needle through the lung tissue to grab a piece of the mass. The pathologist could then examine the sample under the microscope. The advantage of this approach was establishing a firm diagnosis before definitive therapy was planned. The downside was that Barry would have to undergo two invasive procedures instead of one, the biopsy followed by opening up his chest, which they were sure to do unless—as was judged highly unlikely—the mass was benign.

"What should I do?" he asked me.

"Tough decision."

"Thing is, I just want to get it over with. I only want them cutting into me once."

This, we agreed, was what they would do. He completed an advance directive. He wanted to make sure I had a copy. He thought he was going to die.

"Have you got any family left, Barry?"

"Just you and Sharon, Doc." Sharon was his payee, the person designated to receive his disability checks and make sure they were spent on food and rent, not booze, a strategy that worked only so well.

So on Thanksgiving morning, the day after his surgery, I, his surrogate family, sat with Barry in the hospital. It was a social, and, as it turned out, celebratory visit. The mass, his surgeon had told him, was scar tissue from an old pneumonia. Having escaped a death sentence, Barry was in a great and garrulous mood.

"Remember that summer I was so tanned?" he asked me.

I did. It was at the tail end of his TB therapy, before he fired me. He'd been so deeply bronzed that MAW and I contemplated, though we failed to establish, a pathological diagnosis to account for the dark hue of his skin. It was sheer medical paranoia: some dread disorder must be lurking behind every deviation from a narrowly conceived sense of normality. We were a bit like a mob, MAW and I. Either of us alone might have watched and waited.

"I had a job that summer that kept me out in the sun for hours," Barry now told me. He'd organized a panhandling ring with two buddies, all of them vets. He staked out their territory, chasing out all interlopers, and set the hours. Each man kept whatever money he'd snagged on his shift. Barry had done the field research to determine which intersections had the most traffic and where cars were frequently obliged to stop long enough to hand some cash out through the car window. He didn't even mess with the downtown area. He went for the gold: suburbia. He and his pals tapped into an abundant supply of middle-class guilt and extracted upwards of fifty dollars an hour on a good day, he insisted, selling the belief that you have contributed to the relief of poverty.

I knew the story was true, because I'd seen him once myself, miles from downtown, standing at a busy freeway exit. At the time, I'd figured it had to be someone else.

I cringe as I write this now, thinking of the lone men and women who park themselves along freeway off-ramps all over the city with those heartbreaking signs: *Out of work veteran. Homeless. Sick baby at home. Lost my job. Please help. God bless.* Maybe a few are running a scam. Most are not.

Three months after Barry's surgery, three months after I'd requested the surgical records, I finally received a copy. The VA was noto-
rious for such delays. I paged to the pathology report, the results of
the microscopic exam of the mass excised from Barry's lung. It was
a caseating granuloma, typical for TB. Unfortunately, no one had
thought to culture the tissue for TB, the definitive test. But there was
no doubt.

My first horrified thought was that I'd been party to a major,
unnecessary surgery, a thoughtless and brutal assault. My second
thoughts were murkier. What if we'd made the correct move, given
the possibility of resurgent TB, and biopsied the mass first. What if
we'd known the mass was TB?

Option one: treat the infection with drugs; the drugs would probably kill him.

Option two: let the infection take its course; it would probably
kill him.

Option three: cut out as much of the infected mass as possible and
cross our fingers.

Option three never would have made the table. No surgeon would
agree to such an obsolete approach. It would have been barbaric. But
now it was done. Lucky Barry. It might have saved his life.

The pulmonologist at the VA called Barry in to review his case. TB
bacilli loved to hide out in the lymph nodes of the chest and Barry's
nodes did not look normal. Reactive nodes, that's what the pulmonologist decided. Irritated by the presence of TB in the neighborhood,
they'd fattened up to fight it, but were not themselves infected. He
had no way to know, short of taking them out and looking at them
under the microscope. No one had the stomach for that. Any other
patient would have been a prime candidate for more anti-TB drugs.
No one had much stomach for that either.

There was lots of mulling over. Then we all, the pulmonologist, MAW, and I, threw up our hands. Nothing to do but wait and see.

✶

A decade passed. Mostly Barry was not drinking. He suffered a couple of small strokes. He became a vendor for *Street Roots*, the local tabloid published for and by the homeless community. At the time the paper was focused primarily on issues related to homelessness and offered its vendors a taste of success, self-respect, and independence.

He bought the papers for two bits and sold them for a dollar, claiming a spot in front of a coffee shop down the street from the clinic. He'd sit on the seat of his walker and peddle the paper. With every new edition, he'd drop off a copy at the clinic for me, no charge. I suppose the small sales income helped, but Barry sold the papers because he wanted to be part of something bigger than himself, a community. Eventually he built up a customer base of around 150. Nice people, folks who would stop and chat, remember his name, give him a big tip at Christmas.

For a while, Barry served on the consumer advisory council for the county primary care clinics. He was behaving like a responsible citizen. How was I supposed to square that with the notion that he was, and always would be, an antisocial type? It was better to hang onto the idea that people can change, even in profound and surprising ways. Barry was not the person he'd been decades earlier.

When I retired, Barry came to the party the clinic threw me. He sat on his walker in the reception room where folks milled about, everyone hugged, photos were taken, and cake was eaten. More than twenty years had passed since we'd met. He was sixty-six years old, sober, and still vending *Street Roots*. I wagered his TB was licked.

LET'S HAVE A LOOK

I went to court on a brilliant fall morning. The cloudless sky radiated a cerulean blue through crisp air purged of summer's heat and smog. As I threaded my way along crowded sidewalks, rays of sunshine poked slantwise between the buildings, casting elongated shafts of light on the concrete. I should have gloried in the crystalline beauty of a rare day in the otherwise rainy autumn of the Pacific Northwest. Instead, I was fretting about Scotty—sick, starving, and homeless, and not in full possession of his faculties. Where would he sleep at night this winter? That, you could say, was the question before the court.

※

Three years earlier: from the point low on his flank where he'd driven a dirty needle into his skin, the ulcer ascended a dozen, ragged inches. The rolled edges of skin shrank back from a narrow crater that oozed blood, pus, and the stink of decomposing flesh. Six months ago, a surgeon had laid open the skin to drain an abscess tunneling north. It had never healed.

The wound didn't bother Scotty. It bothered his caseworker. She'd dragged him in to see me. My job was to fix it. I loved the bright optimism of these often young, always female workers who'd *finally* bullied Hank, or Joe, or Carlos into coming into the clinic and getting that problem taken care of, once and for all. As if I were a magician.

With round eyes and parted lips, middle-aged Scotty looked more like a bewildered child. Dirt was ground into the pores of his skin. His nails were rimmed with grime, his hair matted and dull. He had several days of beard growth and the distinctive odor of a human body long unwashed, a fusion of dirt and bodily leakage. In the tiny exam room, the smell was tough. *Geezus, you stink!* I might have said to Scotty. He would have returned a blank stare. Instead I breathed through my mouth.

"Let's have a look," I'd said. At the wound, I meant.

I was reaching for a drape when Scotty stood up and dropped his filthy jeans and raised his shirt. He wore no underwear. It was awkward, this timid man standing half-naked in front of two women. I invited him to sit on the exam table and spread the paper sheet over his lap. His jeans bunched down around his ankles, the fabric stiff with dried gunk where the pants had rubbed against the open wound.

Lots of the folks who found their way to Burnside Health Center lived in a park, under a bridge, or curled up in a doorway. Still, they would find a run of cold water, a free shower, the shelter with a laundry room. The men shaved their chins, the women their legs. They talked a pal into clipping their hair and pared down their nails with a pocket knife. In their packs and pockets they carried toothbrushes. At Christmas, along with gloves and hats and socks, the clinic gifted bags of toothpaste, deodorant, razors, and shampoo to grateful patients. Keeping clean was one way to hang on to dignity.

When a patient appeared in the clinic in Scotty's state, something beyond the demands of street living was at work—some problem severe enough to blot out the desire for social acceptance and the natural aversion to bodily contamination and rot, some disorder so terrible it rendered a person insensible even to the discomforts of personal soiling; the stink of their pits, crotch, and feet; the sour taste of their mouths; the chafe of their dirt-stiff clothes. Those who were unclean suffered conditions that were grave and unrelenting, usually some combination of mental illness and intellectual disability. Or late stage substance abuse. Or all of it together.

Scotty was diagnosed with schizophrenia. He was not homeless, not yet. But he was out on the street a lot. Over the next three years, during which I would fail to heal the wound, I would periodically spot him on a downtown corner. Always standing, never moving, gaunt and disheveled, hands loose at his side. Foot traffic would flow around him as he rotated his head from side to side with a baffled expression. He always looked lost. Once or twice he gazed straight at me, his face blank, as if I were a stranger. I never approached him on the street and maybe that was a mistake. Scotty didn't invite me into his world and I didn't want to intrude, make him think I was following him or keeping tabs. But why would he think that? Maybe he'd take a friendly hello on the street at face value. Perhaps I was the more paranoid about potentially awkward encounters.

With a gloved hand I pressed at the flesh surrounding Scotty's wound. It wasn't red or hot. He didn't flinch. "Looks nasty," I said. "Bother you?"

"Uh-uh."

"Hurt?"

He shook his head.

"Long time to have a wound like that. Looks like your pants rub on it. That doesn't bug you either?"

Another head shake.

"How do you feel?"

"Fine."

"No fevers, no sick feelings?"

"No."

"Are you shooting up?" Of course he was. I thought he might be shooting straight into the ulcer. I wanted to know if he'd cop to it.

"I quit."

Like when? That morning? "Good." I peeled off my gloves. "I'm thinking we should get this to heal up. The nurse can clean it up for you. But to heal, it's got to stay clean and it can't be rubbing on your pants."

"Okay," he said, with the same vacant expression on his face.

He needed to shower every day, keep a fresh dressing on the wound, eat a high protein diet, put on some weight, get sufficient rest. Keep regular appointments at the clinic. Stop doping. Stop sticking himself with needles. Wear some underwear, for cripes sake. I didn't tell him any of that.

§

I met Scotty during the time of trickle-down Reaganomics. The US economy was galloping backward to laissez-faire. Medicine was becoming corporatized at breakneck speed. The bite health care took out of the GNP was growing. The numbers of uninsured were not yet a scandal. The HIV epidemic was exploding, as was crack cocaine use in African American ghettoes. Homelessness was on the rise, fed in part by more than a decade of deinstitutionalizing people with mental illness. Multiple personality disorder was the fad psychiatric diagnosis of the day.

Every three weeks Scotty got a shot of an antipsychotic medication that released slowly into his system. He couldn't be trusted to take pills. His psychiatrist worked at the downtown community mental health clinic. Their space was as dilapidated as ours.

The worst of Scotty's problems was his drug habit. He was into skin-popping, or injecting drugs into the fatty layer of tissue just beneath the skin instead of mainlining into a vein. Always he shot into his flanks, nowhere else. A carpet of scars on the non-ulcerated side of his trunk spoke to that. Skin-popping resulted in slower absorption of the drug and the rush was attenuated. Some people skin-popped after they'd trashed all their veins or because they wanted a prolonged high. Or because they didn't want to go all the way. I'm not sure Scotty made any of those calculations. I suspected he wasn't capable of hitting a vein.

Needles were available at any drugstore without a prescription. Fastidious addicts could reuse their needles after flushing with dilute chlorine bleach. Beginning in 1989, they could also bring their used needles to Outside In, a downtown health and social service agency, and get new ones in exchange, for free. All of these practices prevented infections. None of them was as cheap and easy as picking up needles discarded in downtown shooting galleries. That's where Scotty got his needles.

Repeatedly poking his skin with dirty needles led to infections ranging from superficial sores to raging, gangrenous infections of deeper tissues. Scotty came, or was hauled, to the clinic once every few weeks to treat the wounds on his flanks. On a few occasions, he was so badly infected that a surgeon had to cut away the dead tissue in the operating room and give him intravenous antibiotics.

Never once during these hospitalizations, I noticed in his discharge summaries, did he go into withdrawal. He was not physically addicted; he never succeeded in scoring enough dope often enough. How could he? Street drugs weren't cheap. He'd been deemed incompetent to manage his own social security income and his payee allowed him little more than pocket change. He was incapable of doing any kind of work, and he once told me that he refused to sell his body. As if someone would buy.

Most of the time the only drug he injected was the trace of heroin or coke that remained in the discarded needles, contaminated with blood and all sorts of viral nasties. Scotty already had hepatitis when I met him. A miracle he didn't have HIV, as well.

Sometimes, he confessed, he'd see where others stashed their dope and would steal it.

I looked at him aghast. "They're not going to be happy if they catch you."

"Uh-huh."

"What if you get a lot more dope than you're used to? You could overdose and kill yourself that way."

He gave me one of his guileless stares. I had the impression that his own thoughts came at him so fast and furious they drowned out any externally derived stimuli. Like his doctor warning him that his thievery could wind up killing him.

He reported that voices told him to use drugs. I didn't doubt it, but I thought it more likely that he doped in an effort to escape a profound internal dysphoria, that the voices themselves were the manifestation of a mind that could not bear itself. Maybe the act of sticking a needle into his flesh was enough. Perhaps the sharp prick was the reward. It occurred to me I'd never seen him obviously loaded.

Scotty would swear he wasn't going to shoot up anymore. He would occasionally keep his promise for a few weeks or months, then he'd be back with a fresh set of infected puncture wounds, plus that dreadful ulcer on his flank. Sometimes its dimensions shrank and islands of healthy tissue would sprout at the margins, but it never closed. It didn't help that Scotty was grossly undernourished. Maybe he had as much trouble hustling food as he did finding drugs.

I don't believe Scotty ever grasped in any meaningful way the risks he took. His ability to absorb and process information was limited. I once asked a psychologist to test his cognitive function, but Scotty was unable to cooperate with even the simplest tests. How fast could you draw a line between a bunch of numbered circles when some disembodied voice was yelling at you?

❦

Scotty began to spiral out of control the third summer after I met him. By July his trunk was so littered with the infectious debris of found needles that he'd earned another hospital stay. Just a few weeks after discharge, he was back in the clinic with hot, red swellings all over the one side of his belly. The years-old surgical gash on the opposite flank was ulcerated and draining. His filthy jeans rode over the wound, no underwear. He'd never tried to conceal or pretend; it might have taken more finesse than he could muster. But on this visit, he claimed he'd run into a barbed wire fence. It was the only time he ever lied about his habit to me. I think he knew he was in trouble.

Gloomy and frustrated, I arranged to meet with the mental health workers involved with Scotty, who lived at a transitional housing project for the homeless. Scotty, they told me, would show up literally dripping blood and pus, onto the furniture even, where other residents might have liked to sit. He refused to come to the clinic to see me. He'd taken to lancing his own abscesses with a razor blade. They were on the verge of discharging him. He'd violated too many rules and too many agreements too many times, and the safety of the other residents was at stake.

Scotty was not welcome at any of the local shelters, and no other supervised housing operation would accept him. He'd soon be living under a bridge, where he might die quietly from exposure, starvation, or blood poisoning. He would not have been the first homeless person to perish on the streets of Portland.

When told they would boot him out if he didn't shape up, Scotty vanished. Worried workers alerted both police and CHIERS (Central City Concern Hooper Inebriate Emergency Response Service). The CHIERS van cruised the downtown area for folks so drunk or stoned that they constituted a risk to themselves or others, including offending the patrons of downtown businesses, who didn't want to walk around bodies sprawled on the sidewalk. The van transported the folks to Hooper's sobering station, where they could puke, pass out, or fly into a drug-addled rage in secure, concrete holding pens under the no-bullshit watch of trained emergency medical techs. The police brought people in, too, from all over the city. After a night in sobering, those who'd decided they'd had enough were granted a free pass to the detox unit upstairs.

Three weeks later someone picked Scotty up, CHIERS or police, I'm not sure which. He was in such bad shape he was admitted straightaway to the hospital.

✺

The day he was good for discharge, the doctors at the hospital put Scotty on a mental health hold. They could keep him for five days max, until the court could weigh in. Without protective confinement,

I judged his chances of surviving the winter without housing at less than fifty-fifty.

Still, it was a big deal. Never in fifteen years of doctoring, half of it spent ministering to some of the most impaired persons on the planet, had I petitioned the court to lock up a patient. The idea conjured up images of flat-faced, shuffling individuals attended by a corps of mean-spirited control freaks, in a bleak environment where private agonies were subdued by chemical brutalities that destroyed the victim's humanity. It was an image gleaned from the popular media of decades earlier, recently refreshed by another viewing of *One Flew Over the Cuckoo's Nest*. But, I disciplined myself to think, I was not sending Scotty into the hands of Nurse Ratched. In retrospect, I should not have been so sanguine. Within ten years the US Department of Justice would be investigating Oregon State Hospital, where *Cuckoo's Nest* was filmed, for patterns of substandard care and safety violations.

On that gorgeous fall day, Scotty was seated at one end of a large, oval table in the small room devoted to commitment hearings. He was clean, and twenty-three days off the streets had plumped him up. The nursing home reported he was eating ravenously. His short graying hair stood up spiky and undisciplined from his habit of running his fingers through it. The same bewildered look played across his face. I couldn't see the ulcerated wound on his flank, but I knew from the records it was still there.

A patient had to be in dire straits before the courts in Oregon would agree to send him up. The days of locking a person up against their will for deviancy or nonconformity in the name of order and safety were pretty much over. If someone like Scotty happened to die under a bridge, it was a tragedy, but not the fault of a system that protected his right to choose to live under a bridge. I prepared myself to lose this argument.

The judge du jour was a rotund, middle-aged redhead with a mellifluous southern accent and easy laugh. He appeared sure of himself; his presence was commanding, though not arrogant. I felt myself slip into the comforting embrace of his authority. Maybe he was the one to shoulder the responsibility for this mess. Seated next to him was the court recorder with whom he chatted in low tones. On his other side was the psychiatrist whose job it was to conduct on-the-spot psychiatric assessments pointed at the deceptively simple question: Does this person constitute a danger to himself due to mental illness?

Across from the judge sat the lawyer from the district attorney's office, who'd been assigned to prosecute the case. He possessed a sympathetic but superficial understanding of Scotty's predicament. Only minutes before the hearing commenced he'd interviewed me and others in the hallway to prepare his arguments. It was the first time we'd spoken.

The assistant district attorney called me as the first witness. My task was to establish three distinct points and link them together in a causal chain: (one) Scotty's life was in danger because (two) he lacked basic skills of judgment and reasoning and (three) these deficiencies were a direct effect of his mental disorder. Guided by the prosecutor and queries interjected by the judge, I summarized my years of experience with Scotty. The forced recital of his failings was not fun. I found it difficult to look at him.

When Scotty's attorney challenged my testimony as hearsay, the judge overruled her. He considered it well within my scope of professional authority to glean information from collateral sources and bring it to bear on my assessment. He wanted to hear my opinion and expected me to be judicious and reliable in my rendering of the truth. He sustained only one objection, that I had not myself witnessed Scotty shooting up and could not say with certainty that all of Scotty's infections arose from his use of dirty needles (as opposed to, say, running headlong into a patch of barbed wire). Scotty's ready admission of injection drug abuse made the point moot. Scotty's counsel declined to cross-examine me.

The judge announced he would proceed directly to questioning of Scotty without calling more witnesses. Workers from the mental health clinic had come to testify as well. They knew Scotty better than

I did, had logged more hours with him. But the court was not interested in what they had to say. My professional authority trumped their experience.

Doctors are called upon to make these kinds of judgments all the time. Is this man so disabled he should not have to work any longer? Does this fellow deserve compensation for his injury? Is this old lady's mind so gone she can't learn English and should be granted citizenship anyway? As if these were purely technical issues, as if they could be answered apart from all other considerations.

Well, I'd say to myself, if a job were available for a fifty-five-year-old who can't read, he wouldn't need the support. Or, he'd have no problem, if he had a stable place to stay and a regular income. Or, that would be fine, if she had a family who could pick up the slack. But these were never legitimate concerns. I wouldn't have minded so much, being the deputy decider for whatever bureaucracy, if I had possessed confidence that the system had my patient's interests at heart. The system didn't have a heart. I admit, I fluffed things a bit on occasion, if I knew that the fallout from my statement would tear a family apart or send some fellow to live under a bridge.

"Mr. Farthing," the court psychiatrist began. "I would like to ask you just a few questions today. Okay?"

Scotty nodded.

"Do you know what day this is?"

"It's October. I . . . I forget the day. Is it Monday?"

"It's Tuesday. Do you know where you are?"

"I'm in jail. I mean," he glanced around the room as if looking for clues, "I'm in the courthouse. Aren't I?"

"Yes, you are. Do you know why you are here?"

"The doctor wants to lock me up. But I can take care of myself. I don't want to go to the hospital."

"The doctor is concerned about your drug problem."

"I don't shoot up anymore."

Hard to shoot up in a locked facility.

"Your doctors tell me that you weren't taking your medications."

"I'll take those shots if they want me to." His voice was soft, tremulous. A repentant child in a room full of disapproving adults.

The psychiatrist's expression and tone had lodged halfway between passive and disinterested. She aimed at nonthreatening. Scotty admitted that he heard voices, but they didn't bother him. He said he was happy to do whatever he was told. He'd never rented a room before, but was confident he could manage it. He knew where his money was, at that place down on second, he couldn't remember the name. He was certain he did not need to be locked up.

"I can stay with my sister," he said. "She said I could stay at her place."

"Is she here in the court today?" the psychiatrist asked.

He took a slow look around the room. "I called her yesterday. She said I could stay with her as long as I want."

"Where does your sister live?"

"I have her phone number."

I'd never heard of this sister.

The judge committed Scotty to the hospital for a period of time not to exceed 180 days. There was no deliberation, only the judge's efficiently rendered decision. The whole process was over in forty-five minutes. It seemed far too casual, too offhand. I'd wanted the commitment, but only after a rigorous and thorough examination of the situation, a proceeding with weight and meaning. This was too easy.

As I walked back out into the now warmer and breezy day, I wondered if Scotty was angry with me, or if he was even capable of forming that particular emotion in reaction to what had happened to him. I thought it more likely that in his childlike way, he would accept what the authorities around him had decided was best, even if he didn't like it.

Scotty was not likely to gain lasting benefit from intensive inpatient treatment of his psychosis. However, with commitment came a bunch of services for which he was not otherwise eligible. A forced hospitalization was Scotty's best shot at getting more secure and permanent housing. I hoped it would work out. If nothing else, 180 days would carry him through the winter and provide a respite from the incessant puncturing of his skin. It was time enough to heal his wound.

§

I next saw Scotty on the street several years later and a few times soon after that. I never spoke to him and he never seemed to recognize me. Then, I thought I saw him again, decades after I helped lock him up.

At the time the economy was limping badly, especially in Oregon, and the War on Poverty was about to celebrate its fiftieth anniversary. Obamacare, President Obama's grand reform of the health care system and poster child for half measures, was in the throes of a vastly incompetent implementation. The local mental health system had undergone reorganization two more times since I went to court to testify about Scotty. Changes were made, but not substantial improvements. In Portland, police were beating and shooting mentally unstable people to death. They'd killed so many that the US Department of Justice had filed a lawsuit against the Portland Police Bureau for the repeated use of excessive force against people with psychiatric illness. Right before I'd retired, the fad psychiatric diagnosis was bipolar disorder.

Dusk was closing in on a gloomy day. I was driving north on Martin Luther King Boulevard, a crowded, three-lane thoroughfare several blocks off the east bank of the Willamette River. We were moving in fits and starts when I spotted him on a street corner, alone, not moving, staring into traffic. Then I did the math. Scotty, if he were still alive and despite the diminutive name and his boyish aspect, would be a very old man by now. This fellow was young and skinny, his clothing rumpled, his light-colored hair flung out around his head. Like Scotty, though, he looked baffled and scared, yet another unquiet mind in a disquieting place.

HEART SECRETS

The sound was unmistakable: a loud, harsh spurt, like compressed air forced through a nozzle or the quick stroke of a rasp against wood. It lasted as long as half a heartbeat. More precisely, the first half of a heartbeat, when the heart was squeezing the blood from its chambers. In that interval, half a second or less, the murmur sharply rose and fell in volume. It started when the inlet valves of the heart snapped shut and stopped at the close of the outlet valves. When I placed my palm flat on her chest to the left of her breastbone, I could feel a thrill, a rhythmic vibration. This was the sound and feel of blood forcing its way through the stiff, corroded leaflets of the aortic valve. I listened for the faint trailing sound of blood leaking backward through the valve, for the extra thumps of a failing heart. I was glad not to hear them.

The paper-thin aortic valve is the one-way swinging door out of the main pumping chamber of the heart and into the circulation. Our life stream pours across its surface as smoothly as a wet finger sweeps over Jell-O. One hundred thousand times a day. Open-shut, open-shut, open-shut; other than a little bloody nutrition, no maintenance is required. It can be damaged through infection, accidents of genetics, degenerative diseases, or the simple passage of time in susceptible individuals. A damaged valve means a constricted, rough-surfaced passage; imagine pushing a dry finger against sandpaper. Or exiting a stuck, half-open door. It's more work than the heart can manage over time. Within five years of detection, two-thirds of people with severe aortic stenosis are dead. After ten years, four-fifths.[4] Unless the valve is replaced. Who would take such odds?

Lillian came to the clinic for a cough that wouldn't quit. She'd never come in before. She was completely undistinguished in looks. Two decades later, I can't bring up any picture of her in my mind at all, only abstract impressions. Poorly and plainly dressed, pale and retiring, a woman on the downslope of life. A woman anxious to make no trouble, who shrank into her smallness, as if her very presence might overtax the vision of the onlooker. She was sixty-six years old.

After listening to her lungs (unremarkable), I eavesdropped on her heart, usually an unrewarding exercise. Most of the heart's secrets are not whispered to the stethoscope and require more sophisticated machinery to detect. The stethoscope itself occupies a singular junction of history, being the first tool to mediate the woes of the body, the first mechanical interlocutor between the patient's subjectivity and the doctor's learned observation. It was the first loosening of the knot that bound the doctor to the patient's rascally complaints, the ones that were never specific or detailed enough. The doctor could plug her ears with the stethoscope and go straight to the source. And it set in motion the recurring complaint of one generation of physicians against the next, that they were losing the fine art of physical diagnosis, the careful process that employed only the five unmediated senses to detect the telltale signs of disease. It is a complaint with merit.

Lillian seemed not to notice the time I spent pressing my stethoscope to her chest, maintaining my poker face. Patients were exquisitely sensitive to my body language and distressingly quick to the draw—*What's wrong, Doc?* Nor did she seem surprised by my flurry of questions: *Are you short of breath? Do you ever have chest pain? Do your ankles swell? Have you passed out recently?*

Definition of a normal, healthy individual: a person who'd been insufficiently examined. We used to laugh about that; you could always find something wrong. Lillian, though, claimed no one ever had. She was entirely healthy. No, no one had ever mentioned a heart murmur, but she hadn't seen a doctor for years, so many she couldn't remember. At Burnside we sometimes encountered folks like Lillian, who, being both poor and healthy enough, escaped the clinical gaze for prolonged periods, sometimes decades.

I hadn't picked up a murmur like this in more than a dozen years of spying on hearts. I enjoyed a certain affinity for pathology, especially the unusual and interesting. I didn't hanker for the appearance of some poor Jane with a rare affliction. But when she wandered in, forgive me, it was great. Stimulating and exciting. Amidst all the sufferers of chronic disease for whom I could do precious little, all those with persistent mental illness whose miseries were boundless, and all those who'd broken down every which way through poverty and abuse, a case of uncomplicated aortic stenosis was refreshing. Best of all, it was fixable. The diseased valve could be replaced with an artificial one, a mechanical device or a donation from an unfortunate pig. I almost never had something lifesaving to offer.

I knew Lillian's secret now, the one she didn't know herself, something dreadfully intimate and important. Otherwise I hardly knew her at all. I didn't want to tell her until I was sure. I said only that she had a murmur, that a heart valve might be damaged, and I recommended we investigate. She listened quietly. She asked no questions, remarkably uncurious—or uncomprehending. I remember tucking that piece of information away, not knowing what to make of it. Hearts loom large in our consciousness. Most of us would rather shatter a leg or poke out an eye than suffer a heart gone awry.

❧

A young cardiologist-in-training phoned the results of the echocardiogram to me. He was near breathless with excitement; I wasn't the only one animated by disease. Lillian had a tight aortic stenosis. All her other valves looked great and her heart showed no evidence of failing. Not yet. *Good job on picking up and identifying that murmur!* he said. I began to puff up before remembering that doctors still in training often considered community docs morons. Diagnosing Lillian's aortic stenosis was the easiest piece of clinical work I'd accomplished in months. It was a snap compared to what would come.

§

Lillian came back to discuss the results of her ECHO, our second visit. She was widowed, subsisting on her late husband's pension. She had no chronic disease; she neither smoked nor drank. She was the ideal candidate for valve replacement.

But she had an ultimately fatal disorder to which she was wholly insensible and the treatment itself was arduous and life threatening. Imagine: one day you're fine, except for that little nagging cough. The next day you're told if you don't let the surgeon cut open your chest, you'll die.

I began cautiously, expecting to improvise. With bad news, some people wanted you to cut to the chase. Others wanted every detail. Still others needed the same thing said, over and over and over again. But talking to Lillian was like speaking to a life-sized doll. I was telling her something terribly frightening and she mustered no response. No fear, wonder, denial, or confusion. No curiosity. Okay. I set up an appointment for her to see the cardiologist. She said she would go.

At that time, we had no computers. We had miniscule administrative support, a narrow view of our responsibilities, and no regulating agencies with a thousand rules to tell us otherwise. Twenty years later we would have red-flagged Lillian, marked her electronic chart to pop up on a clerk's electronic desktop every week. Did she keep that appointment? Had the report come back? Did the primary doc see it? Did the doc do something about it? We would have designated her a high-risk referral. Bad stuff would happen if she didn't go see the heart doctor. We would have pestered her until she did.

A year and a half after that first visit I didn't even remember her by name. Her thin chart lay on my desk as she waited for me in a room. I paged back to my two prior notes, ah yes, the woman with the bad valve. I lifted the tab over the section where we filed outside reports. Empty, except for the ECHO. *What?*

The medical assistant was trained to record the patient's complaint briefly and in her own words. Lillian's chief complaint that day: "Feels poorly."

"Doctor, this heat," she began, then stopped to take a breath. "It's suffocating me."

She was so short of breath she couldn't speak a full sentence. And the weather wasn't that hot.

"When did this trouble start?"

"Oh . . . a few weeks ago . . . I think," she panted.

It had to be longer than that.

"I get so tired . . . I can't do anything but sit."

"Are you having any chest pain?"

"My feet are . . . swelling. I think it's the heat."

"How about your chest? Any pain there?"

"No. At night . . . I have to sit in Harold's chair, the recliner."

"You sleep all night in the recliner?"

"If I lie in bed I just suffocate."

Lillian's noisy expirations filled up the room. Her heart was giving out.

"Did you see the cardiologist last year?"

"No."

"Why didn't you go?"

"I didn't think it was necessary."

The murmur was still there. Now I heard a soft thump as well, called a gallop. *Ken-tuc-ky, Ken-tuc-ky, Ken-tuc-ky*, the medical student's trick for remembering the type of gallop, circled in my head, like a horse around a race track. The "ky" was the thump made by the floppy and failing left ventricle as it tried to pump the blood out. In her lungs, I heard wet, crackling sounds with each breath, caused by the build-up of fluid. My thumb, pushed into the flesh above her ankles for a few seconds, left a deep impression, evidence that fluid was also accumulating in her legs.

I set her chart aside and folded my hands into my lap. "You have a damaged heart valve and it looks to me like your heart is failing under the strain. This is a problem that is only going to get worse."

She sat on the edge of the exam table, unmoved and unmoving.

"I'm going to arrange for you to see the heart specialist this week. Tomorrow, if I can."

"I don't care to go . . . right now," she said.

"I'm sorry to be so blunt, but this can kill you if you don't get it fixed."

"I think I'll wait."

Until she could no longer get out of bed? Until her body swelled with so much fluid her liver would ache and she would not be able to lift her waterlogged legs? Until the circulation to her heart itself was so compromised that the worst, crushing pain she could imagine would drop onto her chest for some unbearable interval before she passed out and died? Until a rising tide of fluid filled her lungs and suffocated her? Until a ballooning hunger for air consumed every thought, feeling, and ounce of energy she had, for days or weeks on end, before it snuffed her out in a gurgling finale? I couldn't bring myself to describe the ways she might die.

So I treated her failure, buying time, hoping to learn what else she had secreted away in her heart. Why she refused to let us save her life. She kept her appointments, took the medicine, submitted to the tests I ordered, expressed gratitude for my care. And declined, politely, to see the cardiologist. She was unable, or unwilling, to explain why. At one point she agreed—I'd worn her down—and we made arrangements for admission to the cardiology service. She didn't show up.

She initially improved a little on the medication I prescribed. But overall, she was withering. Did she see it herself? People who are dying often get more desperate, either to live or to die. She seemed indifferent. Maybe she thought I could do what I told her I could not do—keep her alive and comfortable indefinitely. Or maybe she wanted me to supervise her death, manage it, make it easy. She never said anything like this. She never said much at all. I assumed her presence in my clinic meant she wanted to live. It was a leap I probably shouldn't have made. Was she depressed? My impression was yes, but she told me her spirits were fine. I didn't ask her if she wanted to die. I no longer remember why. Maybe I didn't think she would have admitted it. Or maybe I felt it was too frank, too accusatory for this frail, reserved woman.

I explored every possible fear, from mundane to profound, that I could think of. Had a loved one died in surgery? Did she think she might not make it off the table? Or out of the hospital? Was she worried she'd couldn't pay the bill? Did she shudder at the idea of being confined to a room in a skimpy gown, observed naked, poked by too many doctors, forced to eat food she was not used to or pee in front of strangers? Did she have pets at home and no one to care for them? Could she not abide the thought of the surgeon cracking her chest open and taking her heart, literally, into his own hands? Some of these issues seemed to resonate with her. None, in my mind, accounted for the incredible risk she was taking.

She had a daughter who, Lillian claimed, was aware of her mother's situation. I didn't know whether to believe her. She would not permit me to speak with the daughter. Some not-so-nice family story was behind that refusal, I suspected, another mystery she would not give up to me.

I was struck by how unprepared I was to root about for these secrets. How to detect subtle shifts in the sound of blood flowing through the heart, which diagnostic tools would yield the most useful information, and what pharmacological and surgical remedies existed for damaged valves—all this was drilled into me. But what about the person attached to the valve?

Early in my career I had often found myself fuming about how much easier it would be for me to defeat disease if the patients would just get out of the way. If they would describe their symptoms straight up, give me unlimited access to their bodies, do everything I asked. It was as if the malady existed independently of the person it afflicted. The less the patient interfered with the battle between doctor and disease, the better. I harbored, in fact, a poorly conceived but frankly military fantasy about the whole therapeutic process, hand to hand combat, as it were, with the patient as onlooker.

After all, the diseases on the pages of my ten-pound medical tomes were presented as entities in and of themselves, not connected to any particular patient. The diagnostic and therapeutic maneuvers de-scribed were uncomplicated by any agenda beyond the strictly clini-cal. Nothing like a suspicious husband to satisfy, a fixed misconcep-tion to work around, an alcohol habit that took priority. We studied abstractions.

When I transitioned from book to bedside, I was shocked to dis-cover how oblique the correspondence actually was between the book and the bed. All the nebulous, distracting, unnerving stuff of doctoring—we didn't talk much about that, not in any useful way. In-stead, there were shamefaced silences, nervous laughter, private tears, too many drinks at night with chasers of self-recrimination, furious middle-of-the-night wallowing in various forms of regret and dismay. There were unexpected outbursts of frustration. Once, in a pediatric intensive care unit, a mug was pitched against a wall and all we did was whisper about it in a gossipy way, about the guy who "lost it," who happened to be a senior pediatrician. If patients' feelings were troublesome, our own were a bit gauche.

❧

Once in a while at Burnside I encountered a patient whose will to live was attenuated, whose life-force was too puny to propel her over the more significant obstacles of life. Or who felt herself to be unworthy of medical assistance, or whose world view was frankly fatalistic. These were attitudes I was supposed to battle. I was not supposed to let someone drift helplessly and hopelessly to her own demise. Unless the attitude arose out of a religious cosmology, a submission to God's will. This I needed to respect. And I did, with a little fudging around the edges—*maybe it is God's will that you have come to me for help.* This kind of giving in was usually the mind-set of a poor person, someone who was intimate with suffering and a stranger to her own agency.

My job was to outline the patients' choices and their consequences. I was supposed to elicit patients' values and priorities and guide them to the choices that best fit what they wanted from life. But what if their values were themselves a product of poverty and abuse? What if they represented a negation of life itself? When was a patient's desire no longer legitimate? Suicidal ideation was never considered legitimate. But what about the failure to do what was needed in order to survive?

A fatalistic attitude was something I usually picked up on after months or years of getting to know someone. Lillian didn't last that long. Not long enough for me to hound her into a procedure she didn't want, though that was never a good position for me to put myself in.

It was only several weeks after she came to me in heart failure that she went to the emergency room. She was admitted to the intensive care unit, too sick to undergo surgery. Three days later, she died.

THE WOMAN WHO SAW THE DOCTOR TOO MUCH

She walked into our clinic one morning, on the run from an abusive boyfriend back in Idaho, she said. She was depressed, homeless, and out of all her medicine. She was taking enough Valium to bring a two-hundred-pound man to his knees and she had the empty pill vial to prove it. She seemed practiced at this sort of thing—getting a doctor who didn't know her to refill her addictive drug.

Carol looked older than the thirty-two years she claimed, thin with lank brown hair, no color in her face, and strangely self-possessed for a woman with no home, no family, no friends, no money. Her range of affect was so compressed that it could not support any but the shallowest of interactions. Her gaze was direct but opaque, not the vacant look I'd seen in victims of trauma whose inner selves had been crushed into a remnant so small it no longer filled the space behind the eyes. I sensed a full presence behind Carol's eyes. It did not strike me as altogether benign. I did not like her.

❧

Lots of patients were disagreeable or downright maddening. One deranged woman insisted on taking multiple doses of insulin during the day, despite repeated warnings about the ineffectiveness, not to mention the danger, of her habit. What could I do? Not give her the insulin? I had a patient who demanded an MRI of her chest every three months to check on a nodule that hadn't changed in years. A fellow once arrived soused to the gills and propositioned me. *I'll be your houseboy, Dr. Kullberg. I've got experience.* Still another launched into a drug-fueled rant so incoherent and profane, I walked out. Patients would regularly stand me up; a few of these same people would appear in the middle of a busy morning demanding my immediate attention to some sort of paperwork, a bureaucratic emergency they'd created through their own procrastination. Not a few patients would lie about the prescriptions they were getting from other doctors, in order to get a duplicate from me. People staggered in drunk, demanding medicine to palliate their alcohol-inflamed stomachs, so they could get on with their drinking. Others bad-mouthed the staff, or verbally abused them to their faces.

I could have complained all day about the patients. Still, I always liked them. I found it easy to look past their faults and foibles, because sooner or later they would open themselves up. It was hard to sustain a fury or frustration once they dropped their defenses. Once they shared the stories closest to their hearts, about the beloved child taken away by the court and never seen again or how they once stood, age ten, between their mother and the boyfriend swinging the golf club.

It was the luxury of my position. I was not vulnerable in the way they were, so I could be as generous as I wanted. It was an odd relationship—privileged, but unequal, an intimacy that cut only one way. It had clear, and comforting, boundaries. I did need my patients. I was only a doctor because of them; they were my other half; they defined and shaped me. They helped me understand who I was in much the same way a child does, if you let her. That is, they brought out my best and my worst and had a knack for throwing my own behavior into my face. *You gave it to me last week!* I relied on them for my sense of identity and self-worth. Without patients some big part of me would have withered. But my need for them was in the aggregate, not tied to any specific patient.

❧

Carol never opened up, never let me in. Her defenses were prodigious. I told myself the more consciously I experienced my antipathy, the less likely it was to affect my judgment. Only an unexamined and suppressed hostility would sabotage the relationship or warp my professional judgment. I was the expert here. It was my responsibility to manage this relationship. I was proud of my strategy. It was the upper hand I was grasping for.

When I saw her again two weeks later, Carol had seen three other doctors in three separate hospitals. She said she'd been assaulted.

"Right after I left the clinic the last time I was here," she told me, "four men grabbed me and dragged me into an alley. They raped me, you know, from both sides."

There were no alleys anywhere near our clinic. "Carol, I'm so sorry—"

"They were dark and they spoke Spanish. Three of them would hold me down while the other used his thing, in my asshole, too. They held dirty rags in my mouth so no one could hear me scream."

In a deadpan, she relayed the details, how her clothes were torn off, her legs forced apart, her body ground into the gravel. I sat quietly and listened, manufacturing small, sympathetic sounds.

I reviewed the records of her visits to the emergency room. The details she gave changed from account to account—the day it happened, the time of day, where it happened, the number of men. Not one examiner had documented any injuries, not even bruises. I asked her about the discrepancies.

"Maybe there were three, not four," she said, her chin thrust out. "After all those times my boyfriend beat me about the head, I can't remember anything. I had concussions, you know. Concussions wreck your memory."

Every visit, Carol appeared with a new and painful physical complaint—a bellyache, a stabbing in the chest, a stiff shoulder. Rarely did I discover a physical finding to substantiate her complaints. Each of them vanished as quickly as a new one popped up. I couldn't ignore these problems, but investigating them consumed what little time we had together. Under the onslaught of her ailments, my reasoned, comprehensive approach to her problems fell apart.

After a few encounters, I started to perform maneuvers designed to discriminate between feigned and bona fide injury. I would, for example, apply downward pressure to the top of her head while she was standing. It's impossible to transmit stress to the lower back in this manner. But when I did it, she engaged in lots of "pain behavior," which was the term we used when patients yelped and writhed and we thought they were exaggerating or outright faking it. We always appreciated a stoic patient.

I never wanted to be the type of doctor who drew big diagnostic guns for every little symptom. Worse would have been to miss something, to mistake a complaint for nothing, when it was the harbinger of some dread disease. Good judgment, that most prized of clinical attributes, resided somewhere between the two. I had to battle a less than robust tolerance for uncertainty to get there.

I also cherished the idea of myself as a nice person, and I envied the docs who were more willing to disappoint. I didn't enjoy dissuading patients from unnecessary, expensive, or risky tests, discouraging them from the use of medicines they didn't need. It was a handicap, wanting always to be nice.

With her unending complaints and demands, Carol strung me out on my own shortcomings, over and over again. Shoved me back and forth between opposing impulses, to do everything or do nothing. She made it difficult for me to be nice. My attitude did not improve.

❧

In between visits to me, Carol made regular trips to various emergency rooms, where she succeeded in acquiring large doses of narcotics. The painkillers supplanted the Valium, the dose of which I cut down at each visit.

One day she appeared in the clinic accompanied by a caseworker from the women's shelter where she stayed. Alarmed by the huge quantities of drugs she was taking, the shelter demanded immediate detoxification. Not a chance that would happen. To begin with, I told the caseworker, I had little or no control over the narcotics other doctors prescribed. And too rapid a withdrawal of Valium could precipitate seizures. Savvy patients, the addicts—they all knew this and would use it to score more dope.

You could accomplish a rapid withdrawal in the hospital, but no one would admit Carol for detox. Hooper, the local detox unit for the poor, wouldn't touch a Valium detox. It would take too long. I did not want to cause a seizure, especially in a patient I did not like, who resented my interference with her addiction. She'd appreciate any opportunity, I suspected, to play the victim to my malpractice. I was proceeding as quickly and safely as I could.

In later years I tried to detox a few other patients who "wanted help" getting off their benzos (benzodiazepines, like Valium, Klonopin, Xanax, Ativan). It rarely worked out. Then a wise colleague of mine pointed out the obvious, that if the patient could scam enough benzos to feed her addiction, she could always scam enough to detox herself. That ended my brief career in outpatient benzo detox.

Hoping for some fresh insight, or looking for company, I referred Carol to the psychiatric nurse practitioner in our clinic. After a couple of visits, Carol refused to go again. It was not helpful, she said. She'd tried all that stuff; nothing helped but the Valium. More likely, the practitioner had ranged perilously close to issues Carol preferred to avoid.

§

A past history of seven surgeries emerged, a remarkable history for a young woman with no identifiable physical problems. She had surgeons' tracks all over her body. Despite her "dozens" of concussions, she recalled the surgeon, the hospital, and the year for each procedure. When records arrived from Idaho, they corroborated her recollections.

Doctors had also hospitalized her several times for mysterious pains that were never clearly diagnosed and never responded to therapy. On one occasion she'd been treated for injuries from a beating at the hands of her boyfriend. References to drug and alcohol abuse littered her records. The one psychiatrist who'd evaluated her noted that Carol tended to "overstate her problems." I loved the way he minced his words.

In twelve weeks, Carol accumulated nineteen visits to the clinic or the emergency room, plus one overnight hospital stay for "abdominal pain and dehydration." Not one physical diagnosis was established to account for this intensity of care. Her physical problems were grossly exaggerated or frankly bogus. But I did not believe she was a malingerer, a person who fabricated illness for secondary gain, like avoiding work or winning compensation.

She was telling the truth about herself in a more subjective sense. She was in pain and she needed help. She might have had somatoform disorder, in which multiple physical symptoms without underlying pathology stand in for psychological distress. More likely she had factitious disorder, the modern, more neutral (though less colorful) name for Münchausen syndrome, characterized by deliberate and dramatic fabrications of illness and injury that typically lead to multiple hospitalizations and surgical interventions. In the case of Münchausen, the medical attention itself is the prize. This disorder was initially described in 1951 and named after Baron Münchausen, a fictional character (based on a real German officer of the same name) created in the eighteenth century and famous for his wildly embellished tales of military and other exploits. Unlike the malingerer, who knows exactly what she is doing, those with somatoform or factitious disorders lack insight into the nature of their problem.

Whatever it was, Carol was an aggravation. She kept me off balance. I felt used. I was exasperated and being aware of it didn't help me see beyond it. Our relationship grew adversarial. At its core was the struggle to establish the origin and meaning of her pain. I couldn't just refer her to another primary care doctor. That, within the tacit rules of medical collegiality, would be a dump. I was a nice, self-aware doctor with good judgment. I wasn't the type who burdened my colleagues with my failures.

The dyad of substance abuse and psychic pain masquerading as physical pain was sadly familiar to me. Patients like this flooded our clinic. Invariably, bad things had happened to them as kids. A society that failed to protect its children reaped a crop of survivors who were dysfunctional, dependent, and enormously unhappy. Carol, too, had suffered childhood physical and sexual abuse. Unlike everything else that happened to her, fabricated or not, she refused to discuss it.

❧

By the time of Carol's last visit to me, I had enlisted the staff at the women's shelter to help enforce a new management plan. I limited her use of the emergency room. She was not allowed to see anyone at the clinic except me and only I could refill her medications. She was confined to a single drugstore. I had the power to do all this, primarily through her Medicaid insurance. I had weaned her off the Valium and refused her repeated requests for narcotics.

This was not patient care; it was patient control. I didn't even think of it as therapeutic. It wasn't designed to help her. It was crafted to work for us—the doctors, hospitals, and clinics. It cut our losses, kept us from excessively drugging her or cutting her open unnecessarily. But she wasn't getting any relief. I wasn't helping her at all. In fact, I resented her for forcing me into this role, as if I were the victim.

Then Carol fell off a chair and twisted her knee. Fell off a chair? Really? She evaded my arrangements and won a trip to the emergency room, where she'd netted a prescription for painkillers. Then she came to see me.

She sat on the edge of the exam table as I examined her knee for swelling, laxness, pops or clicks, restricted range of motion. I found nothing. She displayed lots of pain behavior.

I scooted backwards on my stool. "Looks like it's all healed up," I said, cheerfully.

"It still hurts. I can't walk and I'm out of the Vicodin."

Too bad. "Why don't you try Motrin or Tylenol."

"They don't help. I tried them. I can't take Motrin anyway. Don't you remember?"

Bad doctor. I hadn't remembered. "I can't give you any Vicodin."

"I've never abused drugs."

A telling defense; I'd never accused her of abusing drugs. "I'm sorry. I'm not giving you any Vicodin."

She screwed her face into an angry grimace. "What kind of doctor are you to refuse pain pills to somebody in pain."

It was the first time, in all the months I knew her, that her expression moved off bland. Maybe it was even a breakthrough of sorts. She had plenty of reason to be angry. Life had not been kind. However, it was too late for us. She fired me. And here it is. It wasn't the right way for me to feel; it was unprofessional and mean-spirited. But I was glad to be rid of her.

HAPPY FACE

Doctors like to blame the patients. They make the wrong choices. They eat pork belly and sit on their butts in front of the tube. They stick needles into their veins. They let the stress get to them. They don't know how to put on the happy face.

Doctors like to be heroic. The patients want that, too. The doctor will save them from themselves. It's nice being a hero.

❧

As skin ulcers go, this one was particularly nasty—a volcano of tense, shiny skin topped with a red-rimmed crater that oozed pus and blood. The swelling was so severe it obliterated the bony landmarks on the inside of his ankle.

"Why'd you wait so long to come in?" I asked.

"Didn't look like this yesterday." Roger's smile was sweet and touched with chagrin. His hair thinned out on top above absurdly long lashes and cherubic cheeks, giving the impression not so much of the middle years, but of a boy, prematurely aged.

"How did it start?"

"Spider bite."

Oh, yeah? Spiders take a lot of heat for things they have nothing to do with. "And the fever?"

He wrinkled his nose. "I've got a fever?"

"One hundred point eight."

I'd known him only two months. A pharmacist who'd lost his license for stealing drugs, he told me right off, as if saying it out loud and inviting my judgment were part of his recovery. Standing to account for his own sins. He'd used the drugs he swiped. All his adult life he'd struggled with depression; the morphine and Demerol he filched and pushed into his veins would boost his spirits, for a moment. It was no excuse, he was quick to admit. Along with the license and the job, he'd lost his health insurance.

Those without insurance entered a bewildering world of fragmented care built on a fractured logic. If you were a veteran, a Native American, or an undocumented farmworker, you had your own dedicated clinics. For vets, the promise was little short of theoretical; the waiting lists were long. State-certified political refugees (not legal immigrants nor the undocumented) enjoyed unlimited coverage at government expense, for a limited period of time. If you were a woman who needed prenatal care or family planning, you had a variety of options, but you were on your own for that sprained ankle or walking pneumonia. Special clinics were set aside for those with tuberculosis, HIV disease, and sexually transmitted disease, but if lung cancer was discovered in the course of diagnosing your TB, you had no place to go. If you suffered some rare and bizarre disease, you might be able to access "teaching funds" at Oregon Health Sciences University, although I had the impression the fund was more a concept than an actual pot of money.

You could usually get a tooth pulled, and some routine dental care was available for the poorest of the kids, but not adults—unless you had HIV disease. Or you were jailed, where the Health Department provided a full range of medical, mental health, and dental care. During the early years of the HIV epidemic, people were known to commit petty crimes in order to access the care that came with jail. Glasses? We had one low-cost option. Dentures? Forget it. Inpatient care for non-emergent issues, like a cataract extraction? No way. Programs for this and that status or disease or service or location came and went; it was hard to keep track.

The Health Department filled in some of these gaps with several primary care clinics scattered throughout the city, but I don't remember a time when we weren't forced to turn people away. We could not accommodate the need. A network of "free," mostly volunteer-run clinics took some of our overflow, but the care was episodic and limited in scope, confined to certain hours and certain days. Continuity was a stretch. The outcomes weren't always great.

Patients like Roger were lucky to land at Burnside Health Center or one of our other clinics. We could meet most of their outpatient needs. We also dedicated a small amount of money to fund specialty care from local docs willing to accept steep discounts.

Roger planned on staying clean. But as a pharmacist, he surely knew what he was up against. The long years of opiate overload had stolen his capacity for joy from the usual delights—the return of the sun after days of rain; the sweet melt of ice cream on the tongue; the glide of a lover's hand over the skin. Such pleasures would no longer produce a dopamine rush in his burned-out brain, and how much recovery he could expect was an open question. His world had grayed to mush and white noise as every cell in his body screamed for opiates.

He had prospects, though, unlike nearly everyone else who entered my exam rooms. He could recover his license; he had a marketable skill. He was on the upswing; he was upbeat and cheerful. He didn't worry me. It was refreshing. And distracting. He was too much like me. Too middle-class, too professional. Not the kind of patient I was used to working with.

Looking back, I am reminded of another patient of mine—an elderly, disabled, Iranian woman. I "forgot" that she was a smoker. *Muslim women don't smoke*—that's what I'd told myself, making a judgment for which I had no evidence. *Roger is in recovery*, I told myself, in a reverse sort of class bias. If he'd been homeless, I suspect I would have recognized what was going on. This sort of error in clinical thinking even has a name, an error of attribution, though this is scant comfort.[5]

I gave him a shot of antibiotic and a prescription for more. I told him I wanted to see him again the next day.

*

"Feels a whole lot better," he said the next morning. "And no fever last night."

While Roger's subjective assessment counted for a lot, the ankle was still swollen and angry. It didn't look that much better. I'd hoped for a more dramatic response. I wasn't sure why he had an infection like this to begin with, the kind I usually saw in street people, diabetics, folks whose circulation in their legs was choked off. What I should have thought of did not occur to me. Still, something felt not right. Which might have been why I ignored my rule never to second-guess a therapy that appeared to be succeeding, however wanly. He was better, but not quite enough, I was thinking, while setting aside the question of why he had the infection in the first place. I cultured a drop of pus, worried he'd acquired a resistant strain of staph aureus.

He was supposed to come back in three days, after a long weekend. He didn't show. The culture results confirmed my hunch: a staph resistant to the antibiotic I'd prescribed. He had no phone. The nurse sent him a letter asking him to contact us as soon as possible.

*

A week passed. On a small yellow sticky on the front of Roger's chart, which she'd laid front and center on my desk so I couldn't miss it, the nurse had scrawled: *Found dead. See progress note.* Five days after I last saw him, his body was discovered at home. The cause of death was unknown. Results of the autopsy were expected in a week.

It was a very long week for me. During every spare moment I scanned the possibilities: blood poisoning, suicide, heart attack, reaction to his new antidepressant. And drug overdose, it finally occurred to me. At night I lay awake as all reason fled before the pathos of wee-hour paranoia. It was the wrong time to think about anything.

He must have been sicker than I thought. I must have prescribed too much of the new medicine. I must have done something wrong. I know I killed him. His family will hate me. They will sue me and I will be professionally humiliated. His death will be on me forever. It was the anticipatory shame at having violated the exhortation to first do no harm.

Then for brief moments every day I hated myself for caring more about my possible role in his death than the fact of it—too soon, too young.

Hypothesis: whatever bad happened to my patients could always be traced back to some failure of mine.

Corollary: if I do my job perfectly, my patients will never suffer or die.

It was a conceit to imagine that I wielded so much power in my patients' lives. It was, even more, an odd take for someone who believes that disease and disability in vast measure result from the insults of society: soul-numbing work or no work at all, an over-processed and nutritionally depleted food supply, environmental toxins, gun culture violence, living with the grinding stress of racism—you name it. The depredations of society, as we used to say about the numbers of bacteria under the microscope in a sample of infected urine, are too numerous to count.

And my work? It was at the margin, rear guard, Band-Aid, or worse—part of what enabled things to stay the way they were. I was part of a nether system to tamp everything down and cover it over at the dark and dirty bottom of the social heap. I was the crumb tossed to the poor to keep them from embarrassing everyone else by starving to death, perishing of blood poisoning or exposure in the streets. Or clogging up the emergency rooms with their neglected conditions, jacking up costs for everyone else with their uncompensated care. Or more alarming yet, mounting protests with angry testimony at polite hearings, or with crowds of marching, pissed-off people, refusing to cooperate, disturbing the peace, disrupting the order. Demanding the whole loaf.

But, the mind is a wondrous thing. It can refuse to see what it does not want to see. It can hold two opposing positions at once.

§

The coroner found lethal levels of cocaine and heroin in Roger's blood. Likely unintentional; nothing suggested suicide. The internal organs looked good, no evidence for blood poisoning. By the way, she added over the phone, the ulcer on his ankle appeared to be healing well—the ulcer that had bloomed where he'd shot drugs into a vein. Roger hadn't come in sooner with his infection, because he expected I would see through his spidery story, that I would force him to confront his failure, that I would impose myself between him and his only source of pleasure. It must have been an odd sort of relief for him that I failed to see what was happening.

My initial reaction was relief (I hadn't killed him), followed by dismay (such a sad end to a sad life), and then anger. How dare he throw his life away so carelessly, leaving me to wonder if I were responsible?

His sister called that same morning. She wondered about the letter advising him he was taking the wrong antibiotic. Not that it mattered; he hadn't taken a single dose. Not one. She had hoped Roger had died of blood poisoning, as fiercely as I had hoped he had not. For her, a natural cause of death would have been easier to live with than the idea that her brother had succumbed to his addiction.

Had I realized, maybe I could have swooped in, white coat flying out like a cape, and stopped him from shooting up. Then again, Roger knew what he was doing and wasn't about to let that nice doctor of his get in his way. He wasn't even taking the antibiotics—so much for my influence over his behavior. Of course, this was the easiest way for me to think about it, that my mistake, my failure to recognize his relapse, didn't matter in the end. Because it was tough to contemplate my fallibility, that I could screw up and a patient would be injured or even die. Thinking too hard down those lines would have driven me out of medicine long before I finally did give up. And what about the outside world, the one that shamed and marginalized Roger, granted him few options and no forgiveness, abandoned him pretty much to his own devices?

Perhaps this impulse of mine to lay blame at a single doorstep is wrong-headed. Roger and I were in it together—in that year, in that place, under that set of social pressures, constraints, and mores. We colluded in maintaining the myth of clean-and-sober Roger, I blind and happy, he desperate and duplicitous. Failure was everywhere. He was the one who paid for it.

GET REAL

I squinted and tilted my head. "You are taking your pills, right?" The blood pressure pills, I meant. His blood pressure was way too high.

"Yes." Lawrence made a circle with his chin and smiled broadly, wrinkling his blue-tinged upper lip against the clear tubing that sent prongs up into each nostril. The tube forged a double green highway up over both pale cheeks, looped around his ears, then draped down over his shoulders and joined in front of his heart, which was plugging away a wee bit too fast. From there a single tube snaked around behind his motorized wheelchair to an industrial green oxygen tank parked in a slot at the back.

Such a sweetheart he was. A barrel of a man, the buttons on his shirt strained to popping from too much stagnant, useless air trapped in his nearly useless lungs. No meat on his legs, just fluid from the knees down, the skin stretched taut, purple, and shiny. My thumb pressed into it left a dent. Despite all that diuretic he was supposed to be taking. No hair on those legs anymore, but there had been, you could tell from the white pelt on his chest.

Lawrence was a blue bloater, as we used to call these guys, a subtype of chronic lung disease. A pink puffer was sensitive to the abnormal levels of gases in the blood and panted to drive the oxygen up and the carbon dioxide down. A blue bloater was neither so sensitive nor industrious. He let the gases slide in the wrong direction. In fact, give a blue bloater too much oxygen and he got even lazier. He might even let the carbon dioxide rise to toxic levels. I'm implying it was

Lawrence's fault, and it was not. You could take Lawrence to task for the cigarettes he failed to give up after Uncle Sam got him addicted during the Korean War, but not the peculiarities of his respiratory physiology. He didn't smoke anymore.

Lawrence's flabby heart was failing from the strain of his bad lungs. I had his kidneys to consider as well, and the heartiness of his cerebral circulation. I had lots of reasons to be wigged out about his blood pressure. 180/110. 176/102. 192/118. Was he taking his meds? Of course, he always told me. Including all five of his blood pressure pills. Three-quarters of the drugs he was taking were unknown at the time I started medical school. Back then, a guy like Lawrence would have been long dead. The medicines mattered.

I'd been part of not a few backroom discussions with docs and nurse practitioners about compliance, one of the words we used for following the practitioner's (formerly doctor's) orders.

"Patients are never compliant. You just think they are."

"That's not the point. They don't come to us to follow orders."

"They need to believe in what we're doing. They need to understand if they're going to be compliant."

"I call it adherent."

"Like sticky?"

"Adherent is not a better word than compliant. It's a negotiation, between you and the patient."

"They're not patients. They're not just sitting around waiting for our orders."

"They're customers."

"No. I'm sorry. I am not a commodity that they have purchased. This is a relationship, between doctor and patient."

"Client."

"Provider."

"Okay, provider and client."

"It's a negotiation."

"Excuse me, sir, are you negotiating your medicines?"

"Not if they don't have the money to buy them."

"They buy their cigarettes, right?"

"Not to mention their booze."

"Why not their medicines? They're making choices."

"Notice how they never run out of their Vicodin?"

"Maybe there's a lesson there."

"I don't think choice is a concept that applies very well."

"They're not passive. They're not just victims."

"Nonsense. Half of them just want to be told what to do."

"You know, if our clients don't follow through with what's best for them, it's our fault. It's because we did a lousy job coaching or explaining or listening or compromising. Or facilitating."

"My fault their SSI check didn't come?"

"If their check doesn't come and they are out of medicine and can't afford the co-pay and know what the consequences of missing the medicine are, because you've told them in language they understand, and they've agreed to it, they will call you and you will arrange for them to get some bridging doses for free at our pharmacy."

"Get real."

"Look, we don't even know when our patients aren't taking their meds, because we don't ask. We don't have time. We forget. They distract us with their ten other problems."

"So have them come in and see the nurse and she can do a pill count. Call the pharmacy."

"They don't want to come see the nurse. It's a hassle; they don't have the bus fare."

"It gets in the way of their doping."

"People make choices."

Or they have no choice. One time a pharmacy snafu meant that Lawrence would have to go the weekend without the breathing medicine he so desperately needed. I remember it had something to do with who was going to pay, or not, for said medicine. Somehow we managed a work-around; our pharmacists were wonderful, our best allies. At the county clinics, we were very good at the work-around. I was able to pick up the medicine and run it out to his one-bedroom apartment about a mile away. This visit did not count toward my productivity goal.

Lawrence was happy to come see the nurse. He did everything we had agreed on. Negotiated, I mean. Even so I was adding one drug on top of another, after looking for and finding no other cause for his out-of-control blood pressure, other than plain old hypertension. 178/112. 166/108.

On an afternoon I was not scheduled to be there, I dropped into the clinic, sneaking away from my upstairs office to review some report I was worried about. I spotted Lawrence through an open door, waiting for the nurse who was, at that very moment, trying to call me, about his too-high blood pressure. I retrieved his massive, falling-apart chart and sat down with him. I had all the time in the world. I was cheating. They weren't paying me to see patients that day. They were paying me to manage a crowd of seventy-five providers and make sure the care they delivered was safe, up-to-date, and respectful. And that those seventy-five providers saw as many patients every day as they were supposed to, a number which always struck me as heroic. None of us ever managed it in eight hours, more like nine or ten, if we ate lunch while charting and phoning and never took anything beyond a pee-break. Otherwise it could be eleven hours, or more. If we didn't produce an adequate number of visits, the feds would, and one time did, dock our grant. The threat was not empty. Besides, the majority of our patients couldn't go anywhere else for care. If we couldn't squeeze them in, they would go without. We had waiting lists to get into our clinics.

But the patients came in high. They didn't speak English. They were illiterate. They were demented or delusional. They never had just one problem, more like five or six. Fifteen or twenty minutes a pop didn't cut it. Stop whining. That's the look I would sometimes get from people who'd never worked the inside of an exam room. Of course I was whining. Buck up.

I was once talking with a lung specialist about a protocol for primary care providers to manage end-stage chronic obstructive pulmonary disease, like Lawrence suffered. For patients without insurance, we often took care of problems that would otherwise be delivered into the hands of the specialist. We had lots of opportunity to push our professional boundaries. This fellow, understanding that, was trying to help out.

"Sounds like that would take about an hour a visit," I said to him. Not counting, I thought to myself, the time needed to attend to the depression, diabetes, and liver disease these folks might also have.

"Right," he confirmed.

"We don't get an hour with patients, more like twenty minutes."

There was a silence on the other end of the line. Then, "How do you ever manage that?"

I laughed. With a lot of whining. Though I didn't say it.

Lawrence had brought in his pill bottles. They were lined up on the little table, which had not yet been vacated for a computer. His med sheets were a mess, but they were my mess; I could follow my own tracks through dozens of switches and changes.

I picked up a vial of furosemide, a thirty-day supply, half full, filled six weeks earlier. I held it up. "How do you take this?"

Lawrence squinted at it. "My water pill? I take it every morning, unless I have to go somewhere, because I can't not be near a bathroom."

This big, debilitated guy in a motorized wheelchair, with his swollen legs on his pale green tether—what kind of effort did it take to pee? Maybe most mornings he just said to hell with it. Maybe the swollen legs didn't bother him or he didn't understand how they related to his heart. Maybe what really bugged him was having to pee every hour. Not something we had ever negotiated.

"Looks like you go out a lot," I said. "That's good. Don't like to think of you cooped up. Your potassium?" I sorted through the vials and found it, also half full, same fill date.

"You told me to always take them together."

That was a relief. Too much of one without the other could literally kill him, especially with his kidneys.

Atenolol. A different fill date, again too many pills in the vial. "How do you take this?"

"I save it for the days when my blood pressure is really high, because the pill sort of makes me feel sick."

"I see. How do you know when your blood pressure is too high?"

"I can feel it pound in my head."

Lisinopril? Looked like he was taking it almost every day, but I'd doubled the dose. He'd been filling the old prescription, instead of the new one. And hydralazine? Where was that? Sort of a throwback medicine, my latest addition, it had to be taken three times daily, at the same time, and who would ever do that?

Lawrence looked blank. "I picked everything up at the pharmacy and took it, just like you told me." All eleven of his pills and puffers.

He wasn't lying when he told me he was taking his medications. He was, in his own peculiar, but rational, even thoughtful, way.

Thirty minutes later, I'd straightened everything out, devised a new, scaled-back plan, negotiated over the water pills. Then I listened while he told me about winter in Korea. Here was the unalloyed pleasure of clinical medicine, the privilege I treasured most, to listen to people who were not of my gender, my age, my class, my race, etc., talk about their lives. It was a privilege I rarely had the time to enjoy.

I didn't ask about his breathing or his sleeping or his energy. I didn't listen to his chest or poke my fingers into his legs. I didn't review his immunizations, evaluate his alcohol consumption, make sure he still wasn't smoking, inquire about his mood, all those other things I was supposed to do. Some of them at every visit, many of which I could have foisted off onto my nurse. Except she didn't have the time either. Things I could get dinged for not doing. Even though I was the boss, both dinger and dingee.

A nurse practitioner now working for us had previously worked a federally funded clinic, like ours. The clinic was remote; she was the only provider there. One morning, she told me, they brought in a teenager with massive chest wounds from a car wreck. She did the best she could while waiting for the ambulance. Months later they received the federal audit of their "performance indicators." She got a little black mark. During her "encounter" with the boy, she'd failed to ask about his use of condoms.

A study was once done on how much time it would take to comply with all recommendations for preventive care and screening. In a typical primary care practice, it would consume more than seven hours a day.[6] The doctor would not do much of anything else. When the article was published, we whiners greeted it with glee.

My stolen forty-five-minute visit with Lawrence was satisfying and productive (his blood pressure improved), more than any of the other twenty-minute encounters we'd had over the past year, when I would nervously evaluate his heart and lungs (the problems that would end up killing him within the year) and, of course, whenever I remembered, which was surely every visit, ask him if he were taking his pills. Yes, he'd smile and nod. Lawrence was nothing if not compliant, or adherent, or willing to do whatever I told him he should.

THE VISIT

Mrs. Consonant-Rich-Difficult-to-Pronounce-Last-Name is a plump older woman from somewhere else. In the moment, which war-ravaged, ethnically divided, economically exploited country disgorged her doesn't matter. I know a few things about her culture, enough to make basic assumptions, not enough to feel at home. An interpreter is here to shepherd me. Still, the visit will be like trying to make dinner wearing ski gloves. Misunderstandings, big and small, of word or gesture, skulk in the corners.

I prefer to hear a patient's every word, their diction, the slang they use, their circumlocutions and euphemisms, all clues to attitude, education, and values. Where does the patient put her faith, in fate or in medical science? How savvy is she about the workings of the body? What kind of superstitions might I have to work around? At what level should I pitch my explanations, or should I forgo them altogether, because she doesn't want to know? How much will I need to mince my words? How motivated is she to make change? Will she guard control over her life or want to cede it to me? Should I be formal and professional, or casual and down-to-earth? Etcetera. Interpretation makes parsing these things much harder.

Worse, you sometimes get this:

Me: "Do you have chest pain?"

The interpreter to patient: "*Tre donna buoph liin?*"

The patient: "*Au gorda liin, hoersta wampili, cherre buoph, buoph, ne tre donne, ne donna, lenguapelis, ne busthgorme bouph liin sechers, wassentio a babalina a borbalina, liin torme katescequinokele bato, ne tor bato, grimsechers liin bouph yongola, des yongola fremdidi."*

The interpreter back to me: "No."

As if all those other words carried no meaning.

With Mrs. C-etc., I'm already self-conscious about my uncovered street clothes. I never wear a white coat. I don't need the roomy pockets and most days I don't engage in cutting or puncturing that might splash. For the bulk of my patients—homeless, paranoid or delusional, prematurely disabled, drowning in drugs and alcohol, perpetually poor—a white coat will set me apart. It casts a distinction between me and the patient that keeps them planted in their everyday status on the lowly fringe. The last thing I want is a patient to be wary of me. How much this conviction reflects a child of the sixties with a lingering disdain for the trappings of authority, I can't say. It's a choice I make, like refusing to call a grown woman a girl, or not wearing a wedding band because my husband doesn't like the feel of a ring on his finger and if he won't wear one, I don't want to either.

For many of the refugees, however, a white coat is a comfort, a symbol of professional competence. They relax into the hierarchy of medicine. My own refugee colleagues at the health department have told me this, and I believe them. But who has time to jump in and out of a lab coat all day? Later on, when I acquire a bossy Albanian assistant, Ollga Samarxhi, she takes it upon herself to keep track and will insert me into a white coat for visits with certain refugees. I am grateful for the service.

You have only to follow the international news to predict which refugees will show up in our clinic next. They come from Somalia, Bosnia, Crimea, Vietnam, Afghanistan, Iraq, Iran, and a host of Central American countries. Each arrives weary and traumatized, bearing the stamp of the victim in culturally specific sets of feelings, behaviors, and complaints. Wrapping my tongue around their names is the easy part. Reading the clues to their suffering is the real trick.

I don't know this particular refugee's story. She's not my patient. Her own doctor is out of the clinic. He could have conducted this visit with far more dispatch.

She sits in the universal posture of misery, head in her hands, eyes downcast, shoulders slumped, wearing one of those dark, shapeless dresses and heavy hose that grandmotherly types of many nationalities seem to favor. She has a glut of complaints and a mission to divulge them all. Later I wonder if this is a strategy to impress on me the complexity of her ill health because she is anxious about consulting someone who does not know her. My agenda is to focus on the most important problem, to pick off one piece of her complicated story, learn it in detail, map it on her body, situate it in the multidimensional context of her life, and then figure out what to do with it. This presumes that each complaint can be investigated and managed in isolation, a laughable proposition.

I've learned to practice the fine art of clinical corner-cutting. Little compromises in quality that I judge, or hope, will not have a significant impact on care. I ignore what I estimate are trivial complaints, which does not mean the complaints are trivial to the patient, but that they won't kill or maim the patient in the next hour, day, or week. I skip the low-yield portions of the physical exam, stint on explanations, forget the stop-smoking message, defer discussion of difficult issues, repeatedly interrupt and direct the poor patient into the groove of my tightly designed agenda. I shoot from the hip and hope not to miss. I will, I tell myself stupidly, play catch up at some later visit. Someday when I am not so busy.

A few of my colleagues never master this art, and I watch them pay for it with days that stretch past the dinner hour and into the kids' bedtime. Sometimes they provoke resentments in the nurses, clerks, and assistants for the bottlenecks they create, for making the staff have to apologize, once again, that Dr. So-and-So is "running late." Or worse, causing them to miss their bus ride home. They're sometimes not available to back up the nurse when she needs it, so the extra work falls to their colleagues. Their patients either love them (because they are thorough and do pay lots of attention) and are willing to endure the delays; or they get fed up with them and switch to someone who works at a snappier pace. Are they better doctors? Quite possibly. But not by any of the crude measures we employ at the health department to gauge competence. They do resist the pressures to compromise, though, and on my better days, I wish I could be like that, too.

When I enter the room with Mrs. C-etc., I'm already thirty minutes behind schedule, even though she's my first patient of the day and arrived early. Moving her from waiting room to exam room and preparing her for the visit (which usually takes five to ten minutes; Ollga is no slouch when it comes to working efficiently) consumed more than forty-five minutes. The feds, the big daddy in our budget, have shown us studies that prove an interpreted visit takes no longer than a regular visit. And Scotch tape makes a great splint. The math is simple. Everything has to be said twice and easily three-quarters of a visit consists of talking. Those studies prove nothing but the widespread practice of clinical corner-cutting, honed to the finest edge in the interpreted visit. But even the exigencies of interpretation should not add up to a forty-five-minute delay.

Time is already breathing down my neck when, to my opening query, a whole series of complaints tumbles out of the patient's mouth. Where can I get my footing in this jumble? What exactly is the most important problem today? The one that bothers her the most or the one I judge the most urgent? Can I even narrow it down to one problem? Sometimes by the time I make the sort and negotiate the subject, time is up. Today, she and I agree on what to tackle. Or at least I think we have.

For several weeks she's been dizzy and has had difficulty walking. (And why hasn't she been seen earlier, by her own doctor, for this apparently significant problem? Any conceivable answer to that question will finger the many deficiencies of our system and will put me in a mood, not a good one. She couldn't get through on the phone? Phone tag with the interpreter? The nurse wasn't consulted? Her primary doc was too heavily booked? I know better than to ask.) The dizziness comes with a fierce headache that bands across her forehead. The symptoms are episodic, all come and go together.

I hate dizziness. It's a vague complaint that patients attach to all manner of bodily sensations, from simple malaise to loss of consciousness. The underlying pathology can be anything from depression or stomach flu to incipient cessation of the heartbeat—in other words, the last symptom this patient will ever experience if the doctor doesn't figure it out fast. Not that I'm feeling any kind of pressure. Sorting through it is not necessarily simple. Mrs. C-etc. describes the symptom of vertigo—the room whirls about her and she loses her balance. That narrows the field considerably.

Then she adds one more thing. "She has fainting spells," the interpreter says.

Prickles of anxiety fan down my back. Loss of consciousness, especially in an older person, can herald all sorts of deadly events.

Me: "Does she pass out?"

The interpreter asks the patient and she answers.

Interpreter: "Yes."

Me (not liking this answer): "She loses consciousness and falls to the floor?"

They talk back and forth.

Interpreter: "In her bedroom."

Me: "Only in her bedroom?"

They talk.

Interpreter: "On the bed."

Me: "Losing consciousness means that she falls down and can't wake up. Is this what happens?"

They exchange words. I stifle a sigh.

Interpreter: "She takes a nap."

Me (feeling the need to be absolutely sure we are not talking about loss of consciousness): "Okay, let's back up here for a moment. What happens first with these fainting spells?"

Patient and interpreter again.

Interpreter: "She's feels bad."

Me: "And then what?"

Interpreter: "She goes to lie down and rest."

I pretend not to be annoyed with this unfruitful diversion and return to my previous line of investigation.

I know how controlling I'm being. I know how important clues to her illness might emerge if I just shut up for a minute. I'm well aware how unhurried and sympathetic listening can be therapeutic—but what a luxury. Her rambling and unfocused discourse is an obstacle I'm determined to overcome, with whatever force it takes. She stands stubbornly—with her worries and confusions, her indecipherable cultural allusions—between me and her illness.

I take a rushed and pointed history of her stomach complaints, fishing for anything that might connect to the dizziness and, after ruling out things catastrophic, shelve that problem. I review her meds and quickly inventory her chronic problems, diabetes being the big one, for intersections with her dizziness. A couple of thoughts occur to me, which I stash away for later consideration. Like when?

After queries about related neurological symptoms I rise to my feet to tackle the neurological exam. Mostly I'm thinking: Stroke? Stroke!? Stroke!! And trying not to get carried away on my own exclamation marks, because this woman has stroke written all over her diabetic, hypertensive, and stressed-out plumpness.

First thing I discover? The ophthalmoscope is broken, my best tool to rule out increased pressure inside the skull, usually a medical emergency. The pressure shows up as a form of swelling in the back of the eye. Calculating that it would take at least ten minutes to move the patient to another exam room with a functioning scope, since the scopes are fixed to the wall, I abandon that element of the exam. Not reliable anyway, I tell myself, and when has anyone ever walked into my clinic, upright and conversant, with such high pressure in their brain I could detect it in the eye?

Likewise, the tests I'd like to conduct to assess her hearing require a rarely used tool that resides elsewhere, I'm not sure where, in the clinic. I can picture it. Drawers and cupboard doors opened, things rifled, shoved aside, drawers and doors slammed shut again. Empty handed. Cursing under my breath. *What are you looking for? The tuning fork, where is it?* A shrug. *Want me to find it for you? Forget it.*

I'm feeling a bit compromised. When I discover the reflex hammer is missing as well, I perform some silent self-calming maneuvers. Reflex hammers are forever walking off with patients. Or with staff. This was true in every clinic I've ever worked, regardless of clientele served. I imagine people using them to dig furrows in their garden, bang on their carburetor, pry open a stubborn lid, though the hammer is ill suited to all of these tasks. I actually cannot fathom why folks are so attracted to them, except perhaps as a souvenir. I doubt they can be bartered off for drugs and I'm confident patients are not conducting neurological self-assessments. I avoid speculating about which of my patients (or coworkers) pilfer the tool.

I scurry to retrieve a hammer from the adjacent room, in which my next patient sits with what I perceive as an air of impatience. I greet him with a cheerful lie, "I'll be with you in a few minutes," and hope he'll forgive me. We've known each other for years.

The neurological exam, which requires the patient to respond to a series of commands (*stick out your tongue, stand with your arms at your sides, wrinkle your forehead*) seems to take forever as Mrs. C-etc. has trouble understanding my strange requests.

"Stretch out your arms in front of you." I demonstrate. "Not to the side, out in front, all the way. Good. Now close your eyes, okay, and, no, keep your eyes shut, please, and your arms outstretched. Now touch your left index finger to your nose. Your left. Okay, your right. No, with your eyes closed, please, and touch your finger, just your second finger, like a pointer, to your nose. Not to the other hand. No, just with one hand, first, please. Okay, can you do that?"

Her exam is not normal. With her eyes closed she can't find the tip of her nose, her gait is unsteady, and her hand coordination stinks. She looks like a drunk. I figure it's an inner ear problem. (Related to her diabetes? Do these findings, in fact, have anything to do with her spells?) But the more scary and remote possibilities still prowl the perimeter of my thoughts. I'm trying to recall that mnemonic from medical school for rare, but usually fatal, brain stem strokes, the kind that picked off one of my patients years ago, who, come to think of it, presented with very similar complaints, likewise episodic, just days before she died. She, too, was an older plump woman from somewhere else. What is the mnemonic? The four D's: diplopia (double vision), dysarthria (slurred speech), drop attacks (patient falls to the floor without losing consciousness) and—bingo!—dizziness (vertigo).

That's when I remember the case I was asked to review the week before, as medical consultant to a network of volunteer clinics. An uninsured teenage girl from another impoverished and violence-ridden foreign country had gone to an evening clinic complaining of headache, vomiting, and loss of balance. After finding nothing, they sent her home. The following day she died in the emergency room of hydrocephalus. A tiny worm, acquired in her home country, had found its way into her brain and formed a cyst, which obstructed the outlet of the fluid-filled pockets of her brain. As the fluid backed up, swelling the cavities, it pressed the delicate cerebral tissue against the rigid skull until finally, vital functions were snuffed out. Reading between the lines, I felt sure, that if she'd had health insurance, she would have lived. Her condition was treatable.

The similarities between that case and the patient before me loom up, eclipsing the vast and important dissimilarities and much of my reasoned thinking. Practicing by anecdote violates nearly every rule of clinical decision-making you can name, but I find this particular apprehension difficult to banish. It's much too fresh. Do I think this woman before me has a worm in her brain? No. Am I afraid something terrible is about to happen? Like, perhaps the brain stem stroke that killed my other patient who was so much like the woman before me? Yes, I am.

I recommend the patient have an MRI scan of her brain. (I can do this! She has Medicaid insurance.) She doesn't want to. She's afraid of radiation damaging her brain. My explanation that MRIs don't emit radiation flies right over her head. Besides, she tells the interpreter, she can't bear to lie still inside a tube. Fleetingly, I wonder how she knows about the process of an MRI and what that might have to do with her reluctance. But no time to explore that.

Sensing the visit is coming to an end, she begins to assert herself. (Good for her, I can safely say years later. Patients sometimes save us from our own mistakes.) She wants some medicine to feel better and something that won't make her sleepy, because during the day she and her husband care for a disabled grandchild, who requires constant vigilance. Plus she wants an excuse from the English classes she's required to take as a government-sponsored refugee. She feels too ill to attend. It occurs to me that we've just unearthed the actual problem. The required classes are an unhappy burden, maybe always, but particularly at this moment.

Our agendas have diverged. I need to name her problem; it's my starting place. And I need to make sure she's safe. What she needs is a fix. This woman possesses a far more intimate experience with suffering than I. My learned proclamations about risk, of delaying diagnosis, about things exploding in her head, might have little meaning for someone who has already risked and lost so much. I plunge from my internal world of abstract clinical analysis, a bit dizzy myself, into her everyday world of dealing with her problems. I write a prescription that might help the dizziness, if it is an inner ear problem, which it most likely is, and write the excuse she needs, uncertain about how strongly to press my case for an MRI. I don't know how to factor in my own paranoia about bad stuff happening in her brain. I ask the interpreter if she might be able to sort out some of the patient's reluctance about the MRI and schedule her a return appointment, with her regular doctor. Soon.

As I get up to leave, the patient begs me for something to help her belly pain and bloating. I really cannot afford to open up another clinical inquiry, but I get her back up on the table for a quick abdominal exam, just enough to tell that, whatever it is, it can wait. I give her yet another prescription for something to soothe her tummy and advise her to stop her arthritis pills. Judging from my experience with the universal expressions of dismay, she does not welcome this counsel and might very well ignore it.

It's lousy medicine. I don't mean the medicine I prescribe, I mean the medicine I'm practicing.

I return to the stacks of charts on my desk feeling far too exhausted for so early in the morning. I'm exactly one hour behind.

Mrs. C-etc. never strokes out, never has that MRI. It was the inner ear problem I figured it was. In any case, months later, her symptoms are gone and she's become my patient, her own doctor having moved on. She likes me, I'm told. Great, is my first thought. How many of these kinds of visits can I endure? But we get used to each other. I learn how to read her serpentine histories, our time together shortens, and we both relax. She's a lovely person, really, no trouble at all.

My second thought, when she first shows up on my schedule at her request? Good for me. I did no harm. And I managed, at that first encounter, to conceal my impatience. Or in her cultural language, impatience is the sign of a great mind at work. Or maybe she likes a directive, no-nonsense doctor who has no scruples about gathering the jumble of her distress into a neat, however inadequate, package. The kind of doctor I never really wanted to be.

VICTORY GARDEN

Back around the turn of the century, for a few weeks in spring, when you descended the long, traffic-choked hill of US 26 down through a yellow-tiled, soot-grimed tunnel and emerged blinking into the light on the outskirts of city center, there, on a half-acre patch of green created by a concrete tangle of ramps and freeways, spread a fat swath of daffodils nodding their sunny heads at you.

"Have you seen them?" he asked me.

"Yeah," I lied, sensing he had a stake in my answer. I did see them, the next season.

His smile was shy. "Those are my daffodils."

"Doesn't that land belong to . . . what would it be? The Oregon Department of Transportation?"

"Yes." His smile broadened. "But I planted the daffodils. That's where I live."

"Where, exactly?"

"Down the slope, under the overpass."

"You have a tent?"

"I have a bed. And a garden."

"More than the daffodils?"

"Oh, yeah."

"Like veggies or what?"

"Flowers."

Frederick was gnomelike, small and gnarled, but without the beard, or much hair at all. He favored dark clothing, a few shades darker than his skin. Black jeans and a black jeans jacket over a black shirt, weathered black leather boots, and a black, knit beanie, which had a couple of white stripes and was heavily pilled. He'd slipped through life pretty much unnoticed for fifty-some years. He preferred it that way. Likely he suffered a schizoid personality disorder or maybe simple schizophrenia, the type of condition that made a person want to hole up and shun contact with all things human. Didn't matter what you called it. I couldn't fix it. There weren't good medicines for it. I never sent him to a shrink, and he wouldn't have gone if I had. He'd never married, had kids, or held down a job. He had no friends. He liked to have a beer now and then, but nothing to excess. Not that I could tell.

He first came to me to get the stitches out where he'd sliced open his arm, by accident, he reassured me. Then he kept coming, because I would give him pills for hay fever, for rheumatism, for a stomachache.

"What about ODOT?" I asked. "They haven't tried to kick you off their land?"

"They leave me alone. They mow around my garden and around the daffodils, when they're in bloom."

"That's nice of them."

Frederick insisted the arrangement had gone on for years. Had the person in charge of that particular green spot simply neglected to inform his boss? Or maybe one sunny afternoon, when the daffodils were blooming, he did stop by to talk to the big kahuna in the grass department. *Hey, some homeless fellow planted this really nice little garden on our land and do you mind if I mow around it?* Maybe several workers were in on it, had formed a conspiracy to violate ODOT's landscaping standards. Maybe they had no rules to cover the contingency of makeshift gardens, so the workers decided to collude in Frederick's volunteer city beautification project.

Frederick's bedroom, unlike the garden, lacked any aesthetic compensations and would have presented the more challenging problems of urban outdoor living, like sanitation. It would have been a more awkward work-around for the Oregon Department of Transportation than a few flowers. I was touched by the notion that a large, no doubt rigid bureaucracy would bend its rules or look the other way to honor the horticultural passions of my patient, let alone his hermit-like retreat.

⚘

The September 11 attacks roused a patriotic impulse in Frederick. He planted a patch of roses and wild flowers next to the chain link fence at the top of the slope, the only spot in his domain where passersby could view his plantings year-round. I stopped by in the spring of 2002. He'd posted a hand-drawn sign with stars and stripes: *Victory Garden, September 11, 2001.*

"Rose bushes aren't exactly cheap," I later pointed out to him.

"People leave stuff for me. I find the plants on the sidewalk."

ODOT workers? Neighbor ladies? One or two of the steady stream of students who passed by on their way to and from nearby Portland State University? Some of his plants might have come from public gardens or forests around the city, but a covert redeployment of the city's horticultural assets was none of my concern.

The year after 9/11 Frederick announced he was moving, to live with his father down south. The father was getting older; he needed Frederick's help.

He had a father he was in touch with? Yes, he admitted, and the old man didn't like Frederick living under an overpass. He probably hadn't been happy about it for years, I thought. There had to be more to that story, but Frederick wasn't much of a talker.

⚘

The operation was clandestine, illegal for sure, but we carried it out in the bright light of an early Saturday morning. Frederick had been gone just a week or two. I couldn't imagine that ODOT would adopt his garden (and they didn't), but it was an urban treasure, an inheritance from a life lived in obscurity. I couldn't bear the thought of it being mowed down. I'd rounded up a small crew of three docs, a nurse practitioner, and a nurse, all of whom shared an affection for those without homes, a passion for plants, and no compunction about engaging in a little theft and trespass.

Our search for easy access to the triangular plot of land was fruitless. There was a gate; it was locked. It did not appeal to us to climb an eight-foot chain link fence, or to cross a freeway on foot, then scale a sheer concrete wall fifteen feet high, with shovels and plastic garbage bags strapped to our backs. But Frederick had gotten in and out, every day. Somewhere. Maybe that's how he sliced up his arm. He never said.

At the top of the slope, we discovered the fence extended only a couple of feet onto an overpass, an overlap designed to discourage people like us. Or, more likely, those unburdened by permanent domicile, who would want to encroach on an off-limit green space to drink, smoke dope, shoot up, make love. Or throw down a sleeping bag. We tossed our tools over the fence, then climbed onto the railing of the overpass, clinging to the cold steel of the fence post. Carefully, very carefully, we swung ourselves around the post, one by one, suspended for a moment over cars whizzing by on concrete twenty feet below. It would have been a nasty drop if you lost your grip, but we all made the small leap onto the grass. It was exhilarating.

Beneath the on-ramp at the bottom of the hill a soggy mattress was tucked up against a concrete pillar. How had Frederick imported it? How had he kept it dry? Beyond that, no garbage, no unhygienic mess; Frederick had not soiled his nest. The only remain was the rusty blade of a small shovel with no handle, a backbreaker of a tool.

His garden proper, not easily seen from any vantage point outside the fence, was laid out in a sunny, relatively level spot above his bedroom. It was a circle, bisected repeatedly with lines gouged in the dirt to form pie-shaped sections. Among the plantings stood fading and tattered paper markers with strange signs, astrological or Tantric or Druidic or some other mystical or religious iconography none of us recognized, some connection Frederick had cultivated to a more ethereal world that must have offered him the strength and comfort he could not find among his fellows.

The selection of plants was eclectic—shrubs, bulbs, perennials, native and not, the odd collection of a gardener who took what he could get. The daffodils were dormant, or already mown down. We couldn't find them in the grass. We dug up the biggest and the best of the plants to wedge into our own gardens and left over half the plantings behind.

Back at the top we realized, with a remarkable lack of foresight for a bunch of health care professionals, that we couldn't get out the way we came in. We were forced to climb the chain link. Round-toed sneakers jammed into wire diamonds below, fingers hooked into wire diamonds above, straddling the saw-toothed wire at the top—it was a bitch. Amazingly, almost all the plants and their attached balls of dirt, snuggled up in black, plastic bags, survived the heaving toss and two-handed catch over the top of the fence.

*

A dozen years later the victory garden is gone. So are the daffodils. Three of the roses remain, scraggly and overgrown but flush with pink blooms in June. A row of cedars planted too close has flattened them against the fence. One of the bushes looks about dead from the squeeze. It's as if whoever planted the cedars didn't notice the roses. Or worse, they did. The metaphor of roses—in the City of Roses, no less—slowly squashed to death between dense, aggressive evergreens and a chain link fence seems too rich. I prefer the symbolism of insurgent daffodils poking up en masse within a close-cropped, weed-free field of grass.

Frederick's shovel blade, more rust-reddened with each passing year, now leans against the side of our garage, companion to the beans and tomatoes I plant in the plot that runs along the length of the structure. Every spring, his variegated euonymus bush, now more than twice its size when I transplanted it, leans into the sun from under the lilac and thrusts out a golden canopy of newborn leaves.

HOW SAMUEL GOT BACK HIS POISE

"The medicine is killing me, Doc." Samuel shook his head. His anti-psychotic olanzapine, he meant. "It takes my poise."

His poise looked okay to me. He looked like he always did. The same soft, lilting voice, as earnest and polite as a ten-year-old, sweet-faced, excitable, and quick to laugh. He was maybe five foot six and weighed close to 250 pounds. His middle was barrel-shaped and growing, a fatness that accrued from armpit to groin and pretty much spared his limbs.

Of course the drug was killing him. Not in the way he meant, though it wasn't always easy to figure out what Samuel meant. Maybe stealing his poise was exactly right. Though you won't find this listed under side effects of antipsychotics, my impression was that they dulled the spirit, suppressed the vibrancy of the soul. I wondered if that was his complaint. Or if the theft of his poise had no basis at all in a psychic or physical dis-ease. Perhaps it was simply an idea that had lodged in his brain and he had no way to expel it. He had none of the usual complaints related to antipsychotics.

Patients hated the older antipsychotics, the "typicals," we called them. It was hard to keep people on a drug that made them feel leaden and sleepy. Or twitchy and unbearably restless. That dried up their mouth, blurred their vision, or made it hard to poop and pee. The newer ones, the "atypicals," like the olanzapine Samuel was taking, largely replaced these problems with profound derangements of metabolism. They worked a slow con on the body to make it think it was starving. Both types were what pharmacologists call "dirty" drugs;

they were imprecise in their action and generated as many or more side effects as therapeutic ones. No more safe or effective than the older drugs and hugely more expensive, the atypicals were not as great a bargain as they were initially made out to be. Still, the silent assault of diabetes was more tolerable than the feel of cement in your veins.

Olanzapine had put weight on Samuel, lots of it, and jacked up the sugar in his blood to the point of frank diabetes. His blood pressure had shot up along with the weight gain. His cholesterol was high and his triglycerides were ten times normal. Once the red cells were spun off, his serum looked like cream. I was prescribing three drugs to manage the metabolic side effects of his antipsychotic. None of them worked very well.

❧

Persons with major mental illness are:
Twice as likely to die of heart attack and stroke than the rest of us.
Ten times more likely to perish of those conditions than suicide.
Die, on average, ten to fifteen years earlier than otherwise expected.[7]
They often live in poverty; too often they smoke, don't exercise, and eat junk. Worse, they move in a world that moves against them, a world that does not, will not, cannot conform to their rhythms, their wants, their ways of being. They are always at odds. They are intimate with fear, confusion, and despair. They don't get much relief. All of which stiffens and clogs their arteries. Stress is a killer. Then we doctors prescribe medicines that make it worse.

Yes, Samuel's medicine was killing him, slowly, in league with everything else in his life.

❧

Schizophrenia was on his problem list. I was not so sure. What was obvious was his intellectual disability ("mental retardation" being the older, pejorative term). Was it genetic? An accident of birth? A child-hood head injury? Brain damage from meningitis or another dev-astating disease? None of his family was in the picture, no one who might tell the story that he could not.

Psychiatric symptoms are more common among the intellectually impaired, but the association is murky.[8] Does the latter lead to the former? Or vice versa? Do they rise up from a common pathological source? Maybe all of this.

Once I got to know Samuel, I doubted the diagnosis of schizo-phrenia. He was not delusional, paranoid, apathetic, depressed, or disorganized in his thinking.

Schizophrenia affects the races in equal measure. Still, people of color are three to four times more likely to be diagnosed with schizo-phrenia than whites—a phenomenon noted since the seventies and demonstrated again as recently as 2004.[9] During the civil rights era, angry black men were especially vulnerable to being labeled schizo-phrenic and incarcerated in mental institutions.[10] The drug often used to pacify them was haloperidol (Haldol), an antipsychotic in-troduced in 1958. A typical.

Samuel was Latino, a US born, native English speaker, but suffi-ciently dark-skinned to reside on the difficult side of the color line, the one rife with misdiagnosis. Or, it occurred to me, someone, way back when, noticed that he was taking an antipsychotic, leaped to the conclusion he was psychotic, wrote the diagnosis down on the problem list, and there it stuck. You'd think we'd be more careful, but we weren't always. Right or wrong, he came to me with the two diag-noses already established—schizophrenia and intellectual disability, yet another refugee of the mental health system, stable enough to be palmed off on primary care.

He was as docile as a man under anesthesia. I wrote him prescrip-tions; he filled them at our pharmacy, then stopped by every day to see a nurse, who doled out his daily doses. He kept his appointments. He never caused a problem. But hospital reports from years past told the tale of a young man dangerously out of his mind and out of control, at one point tied down to a gurney to protect him and everyone else. When I read that emergency room report, I shuddered at the vision—Samuel wrestled by a small army of men into four point restraints, screaming and thrashing, heavier than the gurney he was lashed to, strong enough to topple the whole thing over.

Like many persons with significant intellectual impairment—up to 15 percent of them[11]—he had what we blandly called behavioral issues. Whether he was schizophrenic or not, the antipsychotic olanzapine worked great to suppress his undesirable behavior. I never thought to discontinue it. He'd been in the mental health system for years; all things psychiatric had already been tried. It was in his genetic cards to be diabetic, hypertensive, and hyperlipemic; a worsening of those conditions was the price he had to pay to be safe, for all of us to be safe. I was not going to be the one who unleashed his violent behavior.

But Samuel wanted his poise back. After years of happy stability, what little worm had wiggled into his head and changed his mind? It was a mystery. He quit the drug. He refused to switch it out for another. I talked sense and nonsense, anything I could think of to persuade him to take something.

He quit coming to the clinic. Over the next several months he fell into frenzies, started fights, wound up in the jail and the ER. They sent me the reports. He was arrested several times. Once, the police tasered him. I was frightened for him—a dark-skinned, mentally ill man raging on the streets of Portland. I worried the police would shoot him.

At one point I sat with him in the waiting room, a cop standing by at some remove. No one wanted him back in an exam room.

"Having a hard time, are you, Samuel?"

His smile was big. "It's rough."

"I heard you got into a fight."

"I had to protect my girl. He was mean to her."

What girl? I was thinking. "I'm worried about you."

"I'm good."

"But you get into fights and the police don't like that and you end up in jail. That's no good."

"I got to hold my temper. That's what my girl says. I got to be poised, Doc. I got to be real poised."

"There's this medicine that might help you with your poise. You just put it under your tongue, you don't even have to swallow it." It was olanzapine, the drug he'd quit, in a different form, but I didn't tell him that. It was a novelty. Did I think it would somehow appeal to him? Did I think it was okay to lie?

It didn't matter; he'd put his mind in park. "I'm doing good, Doc."

He landed on the psych ward three times, each time released a few days later, after he calmed down on the drugs that he would quit as soon as he was back out on the streets. The fourth time they sent him to Oregon State Hospital. Every system had a learning curve.

§

The hospital kept him several months, an astonishing amount of time in this get-'em-out-fast-as-you-can era of inpatient care. I was not privy to the details of what happened there, why they held him so long. The records never arrived. But I could imagine.

I was delighted to see him again after his discharge. He looked great. He'd lost more than sixty pounds. His lipids had normalized, his blood pressure had come down, and his diabetes was controlled. His mood was excellent. He'd ended up on haloperidol, at one time America's premier drug for controlling dark, angry men. The staff at Oregon State Hospital apparently possessed powers of persuasion that I did not. I didn't ask him what he thought of Haldol or whether he was having side effects. I was afraid I'd plant some crazy idea. I did ask him how he felt; he had no complaints. He slipped back into happy stability and stayed there for as long as I knew him.

A MORNING WRECK

I'd just walked into an exam room when the words blasted over the loudspeaker.

"Medical assistance, women's restroom!"

I sprinted down the hall, raced past heads turning in reception, and burst into the ladies' john, several others on my tail.

Inside the first of two stalls I saw her on the floor. I bellied under the locked door into a crouch next to her. She'd toppled forward off the toilet into a three-point landing—knees and face. One cheek was flattened onto the tile. Her pants were at her ankles. Her naked butt, plump and pale, stuck up in the air. She was not breathing.

Time expanded. The moment was pure. Nothing existed but the woman plastered to the tile. Every other thought flew away. My focus was absolute. The stakes were enormous, but I was not anxious. In fact, I felt nothing.

For a second I puzzled over how to fit her out under the door, before it occurred to me. Unlock the door! When I did, hands grasped her under the arms and stretched her out. It was standing room only in the bathroom, five of us plus the woman, the crash cart, and the oxygen tank.

"Let's flip her on three. One, two, three."

On the way over, her head lolled and cracked back against the tile.

"Shit," someone said.

Her face was gray. She took a shallow breath about once every thirty seconds, but no one was timing it. Dr. Rich Houle, aka "Hoolie," peeled back an eyelid. "Pupils are pinpoint."

I found the pulse of the great femoral artery in her groin, conveniently exposed. "Pulse one hundred plus."

"Overdose."

"Get the Narcan." Narcan (naloxone) would rapidly reverse the effect of any opiate, like heroin, that she had on board. (When naloxone was made available over the counter in 2013, so that friends and family could resuscitate their loved ones, deaths from heroin overdoses dropped by half.)[12]

"Bag her."

The medical assistant was already fitting an ambu mask over her mouth and nose and started to squeeze the bag. The oxygen tank hissed. I couldn't see much rise in her chest. It was tough to ventilate someone with a bag and mask.

"Use the oral airway."

Karen Hogue, the nurse, was loading a syringe from a small glass vial.

The one or two veins I could spot looked like knotted ropes. "She's got no veins. Give her a dose sub-Q."

Karen stuck her in the loose flesh of her arm. "One ml sub-Q, left upper arm."

The only staff person standing wrote that down, along with everything else we did and when we did it, to the minute, on the emergency log—except that we cracked her head.

Hoolie stepped over the woman to a position opposite me. He'd broken the top off another ampule of Narcan and was filling a syringe with a long, large bore needle.

"Draw me one like Hoolie's," I tell Karen.

"Got it."

"Anyone recognize her?"

Heads shake. "Nope."

Her purse was inside the stall. I tossed it to the notetaker, who fished out the wallet and extracted her ID. She read the name. We didn't recognize it. She gave it to the clerk who stood propping the door open.

Karen handed me the syringe and a pair of gloves. I struggled into them.

I pressed on the femoral artery in her groin. Right next to my fingertips toward midline, I plunged the needle all the way down to the hilt into the unflinching flesh, aiming for the great femoral vein where it coursed alongside the artery. It was a blind stick. If I'd done it right, I would have pierced the vein through and through. Slowly I withdrew the syringe, pulling back on the plunger at the same time. A thin stream of dark blood coursed into the clear liquid. I was in. I pushed the entire contents of the syringe into the vein. Hoolie was ahead of me, had already pushed one in. Karen handed him another.

The clerk stuck her head in. "Not our patient."

The woman's chest rose. After Hoolie flushed the third ampule of Narcan into her veins, her eyes fluttered and opened. The assistant pulled the bag and mask away. Saliva trickled from the corner of her mouth. She was breathing. She pinked up.

I sat back on my heels and tossed my syringe into the sink.

Karen was wrapping a blood pressure cuff around her arm. The woman tried to pull away. Hoolie and I were tugging her pants back up. She didn't like that either. "Get your hands offa me."

She struggled to get up. We helped her into a sitting position against the cold tile of the bathroom wall.

"Just rest a moment."

She looked around, baffled. She tried to stand and we couldn't stop her. She shoved our hands away. "What is this?"

"You're at Westside Health Center. You weren't breathing when we found you. We just gave you a bunch of Narcan. It looks like you overdosed."

"I don't use. Give me my purse."

Several minutes had passed since we found her down. The emergency medical techs had arrived. They stopped her as she left the restroom. They pointed out that Narcan didn't last long in the system. She could collapse again. They wanted to take her to the emergency room. The discussion was brief. She refused.

She stood in front of the elevator and muttered to herself. The medical assistant overheard what she said: "Those fuckers. Wrecked my high."

We cleaned up, but we never found her rig. We congratulated ourselves. We were a team. We were good. We'd saved a life.

Afterwards I slumped at my desk. I was spent. I looked at the charts before me, the refill requests, the calls to return, the stack of labs and reports to be reviewed, the charts of the two patients waiting to see me. I couldn't get into gear. Thoughts tumbled through my head:

Should have let her pull her own pants up, ungrateful bitch.

My kid used to sleep like that, butt up.

A femoral stick is a lot easier on someone who's out of it.

Can't count on the EMTs to get here in time to save the ODs.

That was way more fun than the coffee breaks we never get.

She's lucky someone found her before she crumped.

We wrecked her high? Screw that. She wrecked my morning. I'll never catch up.

A pity we won't get paid for that visit. Plus it won't count toward my productivity.

Dope sure does twist the brain around.

So sad. She's really got it bad.

Ollga, my loving assistant, reminded me that so-and-so was waiting in room four. I pushed off from my desk and lumbered down the hall.

"Sorry," I said. "Thanks for waiting." He was one of my patients who saved things up, like one-stop shopping. Maybe he thought he was doing me a favor.

"No problem," he said.

"How's the sugar? Any better?" I glanced at the reading Ollga had taken: 525. "Pretty high today."

"The thing is I'm nauseated all the time. I think it's from the medicine. I threw up some blood yesterday. I caught a cold somewhere, maybe it's from that. Cough won't go away and the sweats at night? My old lady is about to kick me out the bed."

"Does—"

"And my left nut is killing me."

I looked up from his chart. He looked pale and sick. "Your testicle?"

"Man, it's sore. And swollen, too."

I looked at his vitals. Blood pressure was 196/112. No fever, thank goodness.

His complaints piled over me, my mind already jumping in a thousand directions, into each possibility for medical disaster that I might need to forestall. Now I was anxious.

I thought of the twenty minutes that ungrateful woman stole from my time with this man. Then I wondered: where was the nurse who could review his nine medications and figure out what he was taking and how and review the patterns of his blood sugar and diet these past few days? Where was the colleague who could look at the sore nut and the blood pressure, while I went to work on the bloody vomiting, the swelling, the sugar, the night sweats. Where was the social worker who could check out his mood, make sure he and his old lady were holding up? Where were my helpers? Where was my team? Too bad I couldn't call a code, compel everyone to rush in and help me.

❦

Karen, the nurse who'd joined in the bathroom rescue party, arrived back from lunch and stopped by my desk where I was dunking apple slices into peanut butter and working through the lab slips.

"Guess who I saw out on the bus mall?"

I looked up, chewing.

"Our lady from the bathroom. She was trying to score."

COLD BONES

Etched into the features of Mrs. Truong's face was an ineffable sadness. Her rare smile, called out by social convention, appeared stuck on, a surface phenomenon. When its time was up, the smile did not linger. It collapsed and left no trace.

She'd fled Saigon in the closing moments of the war, after losing her husband in some way she never shared with me. The war was over, had been for nearly three decades by the time I met her. But her presence in Portland arced back to that conflagration on the other side of the world. For me, the war in Vietnam had faded to one of many outbursts in the history of Western dominion over the developing countries of the southern hemisphere. For her, the war was a watershed event that had washed her ashore in urban America. That fact of her life seemed basic to me—basic to her illness and to our relationship. But for the war, she and I would never have met.

❧

The year 1969. I remember how delirious we were, chanting and yelling until we were hoarse, thousands of students marching on the I-5 freeway from the University of Washington to Seattle city center. We had shut the freeway down.

I remember how pissed off and full of ourselves we were when we refused to vacate the steps of the federal courthouse, and how hard I ran when the police came, not daring to look back, because then I might stumble and be crushed under the boots and swinging sticks of the helmeted men.

I remember how fast the MPs picked us up after we snuck onto Fort Lewis with an armload of flyers for a peace rally. Three of us stood before an officer, whose expression was bland. "If it were up to me," he said, "I'd just shoot you all between the eyes."

I remember thinking this was a terrible war—imperial, brutal, stupid. I wanted it to be over. Whatever my country gained from the war, I wanted nothing to do with it. I wanted it out of my life. It was not my war. And now, here I was, decades later, with the problem of Mrs. Truong. Like it or not, the war had come to me.

I doubt Mrs. Truong and I would have seen eye to eye about the war. I hadn't changed my mind. How did she feel? Was she grateful? Chagrined? Resentful? Bitter? I thought that our relationship would not bear the weight of such questions. I was not brave enough to ask. It was not my place, I told myself. It was not part of the pact between doctor and patient.

§

At fifty-some years Mrs. Truong was only two years older than I. *Looks older than her stated age*, I wrote in her chart. I could have written: *The difficult circumstances of her life have aged the patient prematurely*. But it would have been too bald a statement. Too much a taking of sides.

Mrs. Truong had come to me for help. She told the story of a relatively rapid onset of aches and pains, fatigue, and memory loss a year earlier. Another physician diagnosed Graves disease, an autoimmune disorder of the thyroid that caused a pathological outpouring of hormone. Graves disease could be treated in various ways, with antithyroid drugs, surgical excision, or infusions of radioactive iodine that burn out the gland. But Mrs. Truong felt no better now than she did when diagnosed, understandably, because she had not yet been treated. She'd been shuffled from doctor to doctor. Records got lost. Doctors refused to accept Medicaid. Medicaid refused to pay. Appointments were made and not kept, because that phone call was in

English and she spoke only Vietnamese. Because she had trouble getting transportation. Because the interpreter failed to show. I traced her labyrinthine course through our medical system via a stack of old records. I was doctor number four.

Her thyroid gland was fat and rubbery, her pulse was rapid, and her skin sweaty. Her hands shook. It was a fast and fine tremor that I saw best when she held her hands out with arms fully extended and her fingers spread. Too much thyroid, for sure.

"Man, is she depressed," my nurse said to me.

"I know," I said. Both too much or too little thyroid could depress a patient. But I didn't think that was it. I felt depressed, as well. A saying among doctors: *How do you know when the patient is depressed? When you leave the exam room, you feel depressed.*

I would fix her thyroid. She would come back to me and she wouldn't feel any better. I knew it already.

§

"How are you feeling?" I asked.

Five months had passed and Mrs. Truong's thyroid tests had normalized. She wore a plain, navy blue dress and low-heeled pumps. The young woman who interpreted wore a white blouse fastened at the neck, a slim-cut, dark skirt of modest length, and the same low-heeled pumps. Their backs did not touch their chairs. They leaned forward, rigid and attentive, as if to aim themselves at me.

The interpreter posed my question to Mrs. Truong, then replied back in English.

"She feels tired inside and her bones are cold."

Cold bones. Impossible. Yet, how miserable it must have been to suffer a chill in such a deep and inaccessible place.

Mrs. Truong interjected a few more sentences. "She feels dizzy behind her eyes. There is a buzzing in her chest, and the left side of her body is swollen. Her left arm especially hurts and doesn't work right." Mrs. Truong ran her hand from her neck down to the fingers of her left hand which she grasped and wiggled back and forth.

"Anything else?"

"She is tired and her sleep is no good."

The pain in her arm seemed the most promising, something I might get a grip on.

"Has she ever injured her arm or neck?"

"She had a bad fall back in her country many years ago."

"Did she injure her neck or shoulder?"

Mrs. Truong and the interpreter talked back and forth. "Her neck is all better now."

"Okay. Does her arm feel weak?"

The young woman nodded. "The whole left side of her body feels numb and swollen. Her eyes feel numb."

Mrs. Truong placed the palm of her hand on her brow as the interpreter spoke.

"It hurts her forehead, there, where she is showing you."

"What seems to bring the pain on?"

"The arm hurts when she goes outside."

"Does it bother her when she uses it, like lifting a bag of groceries?"

"She doesn't carry the groceries. Her daughter does the shopping."

"Does it hurt more when she tries to lift something heavy?"

"She says the pain is very deep."

I had more questions. They didn't help. *If you don't know what's wrong with the patient by the time you've finished talking, all your exams and tests probably won't help.* My father told me that, after his decades of general practice. I hoped to find something on exam. I didn't think I would. I asked her to undress to the waist and gave her a flimsy paper drape.

On examination: Her tremor and tachycardia were gone. She had no deformities or wasting. She winced when I touched certain spots around her shoulder, but they didn't correspond to the anatomical structures that interested me. I raised my arm, touched the back of my head, and the back of my waist and watched as she repeated my movements. No problem there. I performed maneuvers to detect a tendonitis. No luck, as if good luck would be to find something wrong.

I located the taut strand of the bicep tendon at the elbow, depressed it with my thumb, and tapped my thumbnail with the reflex hammer. Her forearm jumped. Same with the other two deep tendon reflexes of the arm. Normal. I tested her strength, her ability to flex, extend, and grip. Her effort was poor. Still I felt confident she had no unusual weakness. I poked her with a tiny, flexible length of plastic, which she couldn't seem to feel at all. Not anywhere. No one had a neurological hook-up like that.

It used to bother me how I tossed out little bits of a patient's story—the cold bones, the buzz in the chest, the numb eyes, the anatomically incorrect sensations—as if they were trivial or meaningless details of an overelaborated plot. That was before I realized it was my job to pare down the patient's complaints, or translate them, into something that made sense to me. I was obliged to work within the model of western scientific medicine and like all ideological constructs, it admitted only certain ways of thinking. Not all stories fit. Which was not to say that the way Mrs. Truong constructed her distress was untrue or invalid. It was simply incongruous with my ways of thinking. But what remained, after the translating and paring down, amounted to no more than a few pages torn from a book, from which I had to divine the entire narrative.

One thing I knew. Her trouble was not Graves disease. Not now. I was convinced that she was suffering the overwhelming sorrow that attended the loss of family, friends, and homeland, everything and everyone she once knew and cherished.

Her body had offered up a complex of symptoms, her hyperthyroidism, onto which she could project her sadness. So when her physiological problem was corrected, her symptoms remained. Either they were never wholly related to her thyroid to begin with or they had not yet outlived their usefulness.

As I sat opposite her in the exam room with the interpreter interposed diagonally between us, I couldn't help but think of how my country had trampled on hers. At times the whole crushing weight of that imperial past seemed to collapse into an ironic presence between us. Here we were, thrust together by that history. I felt as if I owed her.

Still, our relationship was destined to play out more on my terms than hers. No amount of conscious observance on my part could alter that. My evaluation and management of her illness was rooted in my language, my belief system, and confined within the limits of Western scientific medicine. It did not matter that Mrs. Truong likely viewed her access to an American doctor a great privilege. I did not, and I could not, help her to feel better.

I had opposed the war. I never wanted those horrors visited on the people of Vietnam. I thought resentfully about Robert McNamara. I wanted him, instead of me, to be forced to witness this suffering.

✼

I asked Mrs. Truong's daughter to accompany her to the clinic. Mrs. Bui was petite and fine featured. Her hair was glossy black and cut into a fashionable bob. She wore a scarlet turtleneck sweater, tightly fit blue jeans with a crease, no socks, and shiny high heels. Her mother sat like a blown-up picture of herself propped up in the seat of the chair.

"Coming to a new country is difficult for many people," I said, sounding patronizing even to myself. I soldiered on. "Leaving friends and family behind, adjusting to new customs. Many people just don't feel well, physically or emotionally. Sometimes they never adjust to their new home." I paused.

The daughter tilted her head. "Yes."

I heard a tiny question mark in her voice. "Your mother looks sad to me. How do you think she's feeling?"

"My mother is happy. She's glad to be in America."

"Your English is quite good." It was impeccable. She'd left her country of birth at a very young age.

"Thanks."

"Does your mother ever complain of homesickness?"

"No. She's here with us and we have a good home. She doesn't have any family left in Vietnam."

"How about all the physical problems she's been having. Does she ever seem depressed about that?"

Something tugged downward on the upturned corners of the daughter's smile. "She comes to you for help with her problems, Doctor." And why was it that I was plying her with these questions instead of helping her mother?

"Does your mother ever have nightmares?"

"No. Was there anything else you wanted to know?" The daughter rested her hands on the clasp of her purse. She hadn't interpreted a word to her mother, who remained silent.

I felt at once relieved and embarrassed. We were talking about the mother right in front of her; at best it was rude. But did I really want her to understand what we were saying?

"What does she enjoy doing at home?"

Ms. Bui cocked her head slightly and said nothing.

"Does she have friends to visit? Does she go out?"

"She comes to church with us."

"Does she ever talk about her experiences in Vietnam?"

"She's forgotten about Vietnam. She doesn't want to talk about it. Her life is here." Mrs. Bui's face was bright and hard.

"Okay. Thank you for coming, Mrs. Bui."

❧

The daughter never returned with her mother. The five-year-old grandson often accompanied Mrs. Truong to the clinic. Both parents worked. Mrs. Truong took care of the child during the day, except when she attended English classes.

"Your grandson is a handsome fellow," I said one day and smiled at the two of them.

Mrs. Truong's expression did not change.

"How are her classes going?"

"She does not like the classes. They make her too tired. She is too sick to work."

"What does she think caused her illness?"

"She doesn't know."

"What does she think will happen with her illness?"

"She doesn't know."

"Is she afraid of anything in particular?"

Mrs. Truong answered and the interpreter shook her head.

"Does she know anyone else with a similar illness?"

"No." The interpreter shrugged. She was the same young woman who usually accompanied Mrs. Truong. I imagined she was frustrated, too. Or I'd loaded my own frustration into that brief lift of her shoulders.

With non-English-speaking patients, I could usually penetrate the barriers of language and culture with the universal language of sympathy, humor, and interest. But with Mrs. Truong, I couldn't get beyond that polite smile. It unnerved me to have so little idea about the thoughts and feelings of a patient. She and I confronted each other across a formidable gulf of differences. The interpreter's job was to breach the gap, to help us construct a shared understanding, a common story substantial enough that Mrs. Truong might have benefited from what I had to offer.

"May I ask you a question?" I said to the interpreter.

She nodded.

"How does your culture understand depression?"

The young woman darted her eyes to Mrs. Truong. "We know about mental illness, but it is a thing of disgrace."

"Tell her that sadness can make the body feel bad. Maybe you can just call it sadness."

The young woman looked too small and fragile to serve as the fulcrum around which the weight of this dialogue turned. She hesitated, then spoke to Mrs. Truong.

"She says her body feels bad because she is sick."

"Sadness can be a type of sickness."

As the interpreter spoke, Mrs. Truong began to rub her arm.

"She says there is something wrong with her arm."

"There's medicine I could give her that I think would help her to feel better and help her with her sleep."

"She wants to know is it medicine for her arm?"

"I think it will help her arm."

"What kind of medicine is this?"

"It's medicine I use to help with sadness." I looked at Mrs. Truong as I spoke, but she kept her eyes fastened on the interpreter. "But it is also medicine that I use for pain that won't go away and for problems sleeping."

A brief silence ensued after the interpreter spoke. Then, "She says she will try this medicine."

❧

After several weeks, the antidepressant I prescribed had done nothing. I didn't know if she had taken it faithfully (it needed to build up in the system over time). I was unable to elicit a reliable answer to this question. She did not want to try any other medicine like it.

"She says she is tired all the time and doesn't like to go out. Her chest hurts, especially when she goes outside. She thinks there is something wrong with her heart."

Had Mrs. Truong tried any alternative therapies, I asked the inter-preter. Yes, she'd been to an acupuncturist and a Chinese herbalist. Did they help? The interpreter shook her head.

It was time to set Mrs. Truong out on the specialty parade. The object of this common clinical exercise was to parade the patient before a series of specialists in the hopes of uncovering some ob-scure cause for her vague complaints. Maybe I was overlooking something. I knew I wasn't. But I was cautious. Or lacked convic-tion. Or maybe I felt I should throw everything at her that western medicine had to offer. As a victim of western imperialism, didn't she deserve it?

Patients often demanded, or at least colluded in the specialty pa-rades, frequently to deflect attention from emotional issues. These usually fruitless expeditions were not always benign.

🐦

Dear Dr. Kullberg:

I had the pleasure of evaluating your patient Ahn Truong, a fifty-one-year-old Vietnamese female with Graves disease. My detailed notes are included for your review. As you noted, Graves disease is associated with other autoimmune and rheumatologic disorders including [short list of diseases of the immune system]. However, I find no evidence on physical exam to support these possibilities. Her [long list of blood tests] are all within normal limits. She does not meet criteria for fibromyalgia. Chronic fatigue syndrome cannot be ruled out. Psychiatric diagnoses should also be considered.

I would recommend therapeutic trials of [medium length list of every therapeutic approach I had already tried].

Please do not hesitate to send her back for further evaluation if her symptoms do not resolve over time. Thank you for your kind referral.

Yours,

Dr. K. [Rheumatology]

Voicemail:

This is Dr. M. [Neurosurgery], regarding your patient, Ahn Truong. The abnormal finding on MRI of her neck is most certainly an incidental finding and has nothing to do with her arm pain. Please send these patients to physical therapy first and refer them on to me only if they don't get better.

I didn't like his tone. He was right though; I'd wasted his time. But I was disinclined to send patients to physical therapy when I didn't know what was going on. The insurance companies didn't like it either. Dutifully, or desperately, I assigned Mrs. Truong a diagnosis for her arm pain. That is, I made one up, and sent her off to physical therapy. The therapy did not help.

Hospital discharge summary:

Mrs. Truong is a fifty-one-year-old Vietnamese female with history of well-controlled Graves disease, who was referred by her primary care provider to cardiology for evaluation of atypical chest pain. She presented to the clinic with acute, unstable chest pain and was admitted to the coronary care unit on a rule-out MI protocol. Serial ECGs and cardiac enzymes did not confirm the diagnosis of acute myocardial infarction. However, she did have multiple premature ventricular contractions, including one brief run of trigeminy, which might account for the chest pain she has been experiencing. A trial of beta blockade was initiated. Cardiology will follow up in two weeks' time.

What?! I got the cardiology clinic note and read it carefully. I talked with the patient and the interpreter. A miscommunication had occurred. Her chronic and atypical chest pain was misinterpreted as acute and unstable—cardio-speak for: *This could be a heart attack!*

She came back to me with the belief she had heart disease and taking a medicine with the side effects of depression and fatigue. The arrhythmia she displayed in the hospital was benign. Dismayed, I tried to take her off the medicine, but no go. She wanted a name for her malady and some medicine to fix it. Now she had them both. Well, at least she had the name.

🍏

At some point in the middle of all this, I tossed out my last suggestion within the realm of psychiatry; I didn't think she would bite.

Oregon Health Sciences University offered a mental health program for the Indochinese, directed by a psychiatrist of SE Asian heritage himself. I told Mrs. Truong about the program. I avoided words like *mental illness* and *psychiatrist*. I emphasized that they would have a counselor there who could speak directly with her in her own language. Might she find that helpful? Yes, to my surprise, she was interested.

🍏

Months later I saw Mrs. Truong again. She was attending the OHSU counseling program regularly and visited with a psychiatrist monthly. She was taking two antidepressants. She seemed brighter and more animated. She suffered no apparent ill effect from the heart medicine, so I let that slide.

"She looks like she feels better to me," I said.

"Yes, I agree," the same young, woman interpreter said to me. She relayed my comment to Mrs. Truong. "She says she feels no better."

Mrs. Truong wanted to stop the antithyroid medicine. From her point of view, it had not helped her one bit. Warily, I agreed to the plan, on condition we monitor her blood tests closely. I knew the hyperactivity of her thyroid would eventually burn out. Now was as good a time as any to see where she stood.

Mrs. Truong stopped coming to the clinic altogether soon after. I asked the interpreter to contact her about rescheduling. Mrs. Truong did not respond. She was finished with me.

Storytelling lies at the heart of medicine. The patient tells me her story and I shape it into something with a clinical plot, characters, and themes. I tell the reshaped story back to her. If we can reach agreement on a single narrative, we can move forward. We can negotiate, recast the details, add nuance. But if we don't agree on the broad outline, the therapeutic endeavor is torpedoed. Mrs. Truong had had her story and I'd had mine, but the two had never meshed.

A COMPLICATED COURSE

Harry needed a new knee. His old one was shot.

The smooth cartilaginous caps of the long bones had worn through at the joint, exposing the rough, bony surfaces to grind painfully against each other. Gone was the cushion that absorbed the weight of his forward momentum as the thigh locked on top of the lower leg mid-stride. Gone was the slick surface that allowed smooth articulation of the joint.

The knee was warm and swollen; both sides of the line of the joint felt spongy. Because the joint had worn down unevenly, the thigh bone angulated out into a bow leg. Years of favoring the knee by keeping it slightly flexed had foreshortened the tendons. Harry could no longer fully straighten his leg. Functionally, it was two inches shorter than its mate, turning his gait into a wincing lurch. This was old people's arthritis at its worst.

"This knee must hurt like stink," I said.

"Motrin," he said. "I need a refill."

"No problem." I rolled back on my stool from examining the knee and considered the wizened old man. It was our first visit. "Anyone ever talk to you about getting a knee replacement?"

"They promised me one."

"Who did?"

"Veterans. I been waiting. No one ever called."

"How long?"

"Months. They don't give a damn."

Exactly the Veteran's Administration Hospital I knew. Harry

shouldn't have been in my clinic. Not any of the other vets we saw either. They couldn't get in to the VA, because the waiting lists were half a lifetime long. It was the VA's prescription Harry wanted me to refill.

Two refills later I rang up Harry's orthopedist at the VA and was astonished to connect with him after talking to only one clerk and holding less than a minute.

"Oh, yes, Harry. Where is he?"

"He's in my office for the third month in a row to get Motrin. Was he supposed to have his knee replaced?"

"We had him scheduled for surgery and had to cancel it because we couldn't find him."

Harry had moved in with a friend. It didn't occur to him to give his new phone and address to his doctor. Our clerk rescheduled him to see the orthopedist and I adjusted my impressions of the VA.

❧

Motrin refills came and went. Harry was too old to be taking this much of the stuff.

"When's your surgery scheduled?"

"It ain't."

"Yeah?"

"Not going back up there."

"Why not?"

"Don't like it up there."

"How's that?"

"I found me a new doctor for the knee."

A miracle, I thought. How did he do that? Orthopedists were in short supply. "I'm glad to hear that. What happened up at the VA?"

"I need some more Motrin."

Harry about never smiled.

❧

"You missed your appointment with your new bone doctor, Harry. Twice."

He grunted.

No transportation? He got sick? Couldn't get out of bed? Couldn't remember the dates? Had something more pressing, like picking up his monthly allowance from his payee? Harry rubbed his grizzled chin and remained mum.

"The doctor won't let us schedule you again." Smart fellow, I was thinking. An unreliable patient would only jeopardize the surgical outcome. But my job was to advocate for Harry.

I sent him to Dr. B., a guy with a brusque bedside manner, crusty enough himself to tolerate the eccentricities of our patients. A skilled surgeon, as well, with office staff who were kind and helpful. His office was easily accessed, not stashed away in some obscure corner of an imposing institution.

Harry made it to Dr. B.'s and seemed comfortable there.

❧

Harry was anemic; it showed up on his pre-op blood count. He had a rare and slow-growing malignancy, discovered many years earlier. He'd undergone surgical treatment and appeared to be in remission.

When follow-up tests failed to illuminate a cause for his anemia, I feared the cancer had invaded the bone marrow. There, where living space was at a premium, the more vigorous cancer cells would squeeze out the red blood cell precursors. No sense in going to all that trouble of replacing a knee for someone who would never enjoy it.

Harry needed a series of diagnostic exams, mostly unpleasant, and all of which involved trips to Oregon Health Sciences University, which was located on the same hill overlooking the city as the VA. Medicare would pick up the tab. Each department, division, and clinic of the university enforced a different process for referrals. Our clinic supported a full-time clerk who did nothing but arrange for specialty care, much of it at the university. It took chutzpah, persistence, officiousness. An optimism that defied reality. A touch of wizardry. A phone relationship with an army of clerks. A prodigious memory for the intertwinings of a vast institution. Our clerk, Diana Anderson, had it all. Plus, she spoke four or five or six languages; she was cagey about the actual number. She arranged everything for Harry.

Maybe OHSU's referral system was labyrinthine, but the folks on the hill were our best allies. They provided more uncompensated care for our patients than any other single institution in town. They offered a specialty phone consult service, as well. A community doc could call and get connected to a specialist, usually within minutes. The consultants were uniformly generous, respectful, and helpful and not infrequently would pull strings to get a patient seen with dispatch. It was a great service.

§

Harry missed every one of the three appointments Diana had scheduled. She laughed a bit when reporting this to me. She took these failures, this wasted effort of hers, in stride.

"Are you having a problem getting up on the hill?" I asked him. Any of the usual snags Diana would have fixed long ago.

"Well, Doc," he said, shaking his head, "I get on the bus and I see signs, like on somebody's T-shirt or on the license plate of a car."

"What kind of signs?"

"They say stuff like: 'They don't like you on the hill, Harry. They don't want you to live.' So I get off the bus."

"I see."

"I can't go up there." He shrugged; what could he do? As if we all saw signs like that.

A dozen years earlier, long before I knew him, Harry was hospitalized for acute psychosis upon the occasion of his brother's death.

Harry was living with him at the time and had lived with him for much of his adult life. When he died, Harry was in his fifties. It was the only encounter he'd ever had with the mental health system.

"You remember that time back when your brother died?"

Harry swept his hand through the air. "Got nothing to do with this. I was crazy back then."

"Do you think—"

"I'm okay now."

"We're going to have to do something about those signs. They're getting in the way."

"Maybe they're like hallucinations."

I shoved my foot into the crack of this door. "What would you think about seeing the—" I was fishing around in my mind for the most benign, most nonthreatening title for a psychiatric nurse practitioner—"the nurse, our nurse practitioner who specializes in helping people with hallucinations."

He grunted.

He missed the first appointment, but made the second. The visit yielded a typical diagnostic uncertainty: paranoid schizophrenia versus schizoaffective disorder. I didn't care what it was called. I wanted to make the signs go away, so Harry could get his anemia figured out, so he could get his knee replaced, so he could get rid of his pain and stop taking the Motrin before his kidneys blew up or he bled to death from a stomach ulcer.

Harry refused to go back to the psych NP. She and I crafted a plan.

"Don't know, Doc," he said when I suggested taking a medicine. "Is it like the stuff they gave me when my father died?"

"I'm not sure what they gave you. It could be."

"Didn't set too well with me."

"If it doesn't, you can stop it. Who knows, it might help."

Harry grunted.

Over the next few weeks I prescribed two different drugs. He told me they helped to slow down his thinking and sleep better at night. He told me they made him feel crummy. He told me he never took either one of them. He told me he tried them both. Doctors call this an "unreliable history."

Plan B. Screw the signs. Screw the drugs. Cathy Spofford, the social worker, offered to ferry Harry to his appointments. When he was with her, he reported, he never saw any of those disturbing signs. He called her his guardian angel.

❧

The hair on one side of Harry's head was plastered up in the wrong direction, his muzzle a bristly white, three or four days' growth. His plaid flannel shirt was heavily soiled. A sleeping bag was rolled up next to a small satchel next to his chair.

I motioned to the gear. "What's with the sleeping bag, Harry?"

"My buddy drinks too much."

"The fellow you're staying with?"

"Can't stand all that drinking."

It was winter; it was wet and cold. It didn't seem right that a man nearing the end of his seventh decade with a squirrely mind and a bum knee should be out on the streets at night. He refused to go to a shelter. He didn't like them, he said. I wouldn't get anywhere asking him why.

One morning Harry appeared in the clinic with his sleeping bag soaked. Two guys threw a bucket of water on him around dawn as he slept curled up next to the fence of a parking lot. He didn't offer this explanation. I had to ask. He didn't complain.

He took to hanging out in the waiting room, rearranging his belongings and napping. *Now Patsy, if we let everyone do that, we would have a problem, wouldn't we?* It was an adult voice from grade school. I knew better. It would never happen that everyone wanted to do that against-the-rules thing at the same time. We let Harry linger in our wait area against the rules and undisturbed.

Meanwhile, back up on the hill, things were not going as planned. A key procedure had to be aborted when the pizza Harry had eaten the night before was discovered languishing in his stomach. He was supposed to have skipped dinner. "I forgot," he said.

Medicare did not cover the transportation Cathy provided and she could no longer devote a mountain of time on him while neglecting her other patients.

We needed to stick Harry into the hospital; otherwise, we'd never finish this work-up. It was a time-honored practice for complicated or difficult patients. But it was frowned upon these days as a shameful waste of resources. Fortunately, it was not effectively policed.

Harry stayed in the hospital for forty-eight hours, calm and cooperative. The oncologist, the gastroenterologist, and the psychiatrist all stopped by. He underwent CT scanning of his chest and abdomen, extraction of a sample of bone marrow from his pelvis, and endoscopic ultrasound of his stomach, in which a probe was inserted through the esophagus into the stomach to get a sound wave generated picture of the stomach wall (which picture could not be taken around the digesting remains of a pizza.) Dozens of blood tests were obtained.

The news was mostly good. Harry's cancer had not spread. There was no evidence of metastases. The anemia was written off as anemia of chronic disease, a phenomenon frequently observed in a variety of chronic conditions in which poorly understood mechanisms impaired the generation of red blood cells. The psychiatrist felt Harry had schizoaffective disorder, was not convinced that antipsychotics would have a therapeutic effect, and judged he wouldn't take them, in any case. The way was clear for Harry to have his knee replaced. Radiation therapy for his cancer could be safely postponed until after his recovery.

He did have small ulcerations in his stomach. No more Motrin for Harry.

❦

Before major surgery, Harry needed to have a home. He couldn't be discharged to the streets, not the optimal milieu for safe healing of fresh surgical wounds. Although I'd seen it happen.

Harry lived off a small social security disability check that arrived every month. He couldn't afford rent for any nonsubsidized housing, but he had enough money to cover the costs of a few different subsidized housing arrangements that his guardian angel found. Most would leave Harry with little spare change. He liked his spending money. He liked buying a meal in a café, an occasional bag of caramels, a detective magazine.

He had, as well, his own method for managing his meds. He dumped all of them into a single vial and picked them out as needed. When he saw me, he would pour them out into his palm to check if he had enough of each. He was able to identify each pastel pill, what it was for, and how to take it.

Staff at the first place, McDonald House, where Cathy wanted to place him, would not accept the one-pill-container method. They wanted to parcel out his meds on their schedule. They wanted to feed him at set times. They imposed a curfew. He preferred to sleep on the street. We considered a transitional housing project for homeless persons with mental illness, called the Royal Palm, though neither royalty nor palm trees were resident in Portland. They put up with a lot. But Harry was no longer interested and never showed up for any of the intake appointments Cathy arranged for him.

He never groused about sleeping out. From time to time he bought himself a cheap motel room for the night.

He wouldn't be going home directly from the hospital. He'd go first to a nursing home for rehab. We could, Cathy and I decided, cross the housing bridge later.

❦

Harry did complain a lot about pain now. He had no Motrin. His bed was cold and hard. He slept poorly. He was constantly on his feet. All of which aggravated the knee.

A walker, I thought, would help off-load the joint. But even better, for an old guy lugging around a satchel and sleeping bag, might be a wheelchair.

I didn't like wheelchairs for patients who could walk. They tended to erode both the ability and motivation; they advanced disability and dependence. But for Harry, I figured, the wheelchair would be a temporary presurgical item.

I applied to Medicare for the chair. They informed me that he was not eligible for a wheelchair, because he had no address. If he had an address, of course, he wouldn't need a wheelchair. Within a week, Cathy produced one for Harry. It was not funded by Medicare. She was a bit of a wizard herself.

He wanted a pain pill. I gave him a mild narcotic, judging him to be at low risk for abuse of the medicine.

For both the wheelchair and the pain killers, Harry was grateful. It had been almost a year since I met him. We had a surgical date.

❦

"I really don't want the surgery," Harry told me.

For a long moment I said nothing, my face stuck in neutral. I'd been happily anticipating the definitive solution to his problem and now he proposed to rob me of my own hard-won satisfaction. All that effort down the drain. Well, not all of it. Some of it had to happen anyway, and at least the surgery had made a great carrot. I regretted the chair and the pain pills. They were never intended to be long-term solutions. I reminded myself that a reluctant patient was a setup for yet more complications, that misgivings never had a salutary effect on the healing process and could even sabotage it.

I recalled a patient of mine in medical school, who'd said, while being wheeled on a gurney to the OR, he didn't want the surgery after all. The surgeon sort of laughed it off. I was too entrenched in my own sense of hierarchy to object. The patient was drugged and groggy. Maybe he wasn't entitled to make that decision anymore. Postsurgical complications ensued. The patient became deathly ill and suffered hideously. I rotated off the service and never learned if he survived. I didn't want to know. I can still picture that man; I can still feel my own sickening sense of shame every time I walked into his room, at not having spoken up, which would have made no difference, but at least I would have felt better.

Maybe Harry had a premonition about his own capacity to undergo a major procedure. Perhaps he was smart to back away.

I dialed back my own expectations. It was always unwise to develop a stake in the choices the patient made. I pointed out, unnecessarily, how much he'd wanted a new knee. I conceded that all surgery entailed some risk. I advised him that no one but he could make the decision and that he needed to be sure.

He waffled for a week. But when the taxi arrived at 5:00 a.m. at the motel where Cathy had parked him, Harry got in. No evil signs popped up. Within hours, Dr. B. had done his work; Harry's degenerate joint became infectious waste and was properly disposed of. Harry had a new knee.

§

Postoperatively Harry became belligerent. The nurses thought he should be taking an antipsychotic. He refused.

Dr. B. rang me up. "It's your call."

"Then don't make him take it."

But the nursing home where Harry was to recuperate balked at accepting him unless he was medicated. Somehow Cathy soothed their jitters and the issue was dropped. I crossed my fingers, hoping Harry would behave. He did, for a few days. Then he simply eloped, long before anyone thought it wise, before anyone had arranged housing.

❧

Some days later, Harry appeared in the emergency room with pus draining from the incision. He was admitted to the hospital.

The infectious disease consultant called me with the bad news. The wound culture had grown a highly resistant and difficult-to-treat staph aureus. The combination of bacteria, living tissue, and inert material was always dangerous, because the foreign object provided a secure surface on which the bacteria could congregate, multiply, and feed off the adjacent tissue. With a bug as virulent as this one, we had a disaster in the making. If the staph penetrated through to the metallic joint, Harry could lose the knee. In order to preserve life and limb, literally, the hardware would have to come out, and stay out. Eventual replacement would be tricky, if not impossible.

The day after the infectious disease guy called me, Harry skipped out again. I had no idea where he was, but I was sure he'd eventually reappear. Not too late, I hoped.

The next day he was at the clinic, worried about his knee. He consented to readmission to the hospital. Weeks passed and yet another hospital admission. I fretted the entire time, saw him frequently, as much to reassure myself as to monitor his condition. At last the infection appeared to be licked.

Two months post-op Harry still could not straighten his knee or bear weight comfortably. In and out of the hospital, on and off the streets—the chaos had sabotaged all efforts at initiating physical therapy, a crucial part of postoperative care for joint replacement. Physical therapy was how you got the joint moving again. I gave him another referral. He never went. Perhaps, I ruminated glumly, Harry would be stuck in his wheelchair for life.

❧

"Let's get you scheduled for your radiation therapy," I said.

"Don't want it."

No point in asking why. "Are you thinking not to have them treat your cancer?"

"I'll take the surgery."

"You had the surgery, ten years ago, and another surgery is not an option."

"No, I didn't."

"You didn't?"

He shook his head.

"I have a report." I was already digging in the record. I never read operative reports, not beyond the first few lines that identified the procedure that was done. I didn't have the time. I was not interested in what instrument was used to clamp which artery, which organ was mobilized to clear the operative field, what size and type of sutures were used to close the wound, the estimated loss of blood, etc.

Now I skipped over the date, diagnosis, name of the procedure, name of the surgeon, down to the narrative:

The procedure, alternatives, risks, and limitations in the case of this fifty-eight-year-old male were carefully discussed with the patient. All questions were thoroughly answered, and the patient indicated understanding of the surgery indicated. He requested this excision be undertaken, and a consent was signed.

Cut to the chase already.

While in the operating suite, after scrubbing and draping the abdomen in the usual manner, and prior to the induction of general anesthesia, the patient verbally withdrew his consent. The risks and benefits of surgery, as well as risks and benefits of not proceeding with surgery, were briefly reviewed. The patient was adamant in his refusal of the surgery.

The procedure was aborted and the patient returned to the postoperative suite in good condition.

I was not the only one laboring under a false impression. Apparently the folks on the hill hadn't read the operative report either.

Someone I trusted advised me that Harry was not taking the little bit of Vicodin I prescribed. He was not selling it either. He was hoarding it.

"Seems like your pain ought to be much better by now," I said. He was still in the wheelchair.

"I need more Vicodin."

"How often do you take it?"

"Every night, for sleep. Just like you told me."

"Gosh, you would have run out of it weeks ago."

Harry grunted.

"You can probably get by without it."

He refused to see me again. He went to a colleague, who told me that Harry continued to live on the street, never got his radiation treatment, and his wound infection remained at bay. Once I saw Harry in the waiting room, slumped in his wheelchair. He glowered at me.

Several months after his surgery, on a chilly fall day, I ran into Harry in the lobby again. He was walking without a limp, pushing his wheelchair along, his belongings piled high in the seat.

"Hey, Doc," he said and smiled. "How're you doing?"

"I'm fine. How's the knee?"

He pulled up his pant leg to show me. "Looks pretty good, huh?"

Amazingly, the knee was straight, not swollen, and the surgical wound completely healed.

"Looks great!"

"I'm heading to Arizona for the winter."

"Sounds like an idea. Know somebody there?"

"Friends," he said.

"So you have some friends to stay with in Arizona?"

"I don't know anybody in Arizona."

AFTERWORD

A moment arrived when I realized it was time to quit medicine. I remember which exam room I occupied, the rolling stool under my butt, the screen of the electronic record suspended on a long arm in the air, the patient perched in a sturdy steel and plastic chair. I don't remember much about the man other than his race, which was white, his language, which was English, and that he was not difficult—not demanding, disjointed, dissembling, etc. He was a nice man. What I remember distinctly about that encounter was my sudden remove from it. I was not interested in what the patient was telling me.

My time in the clinic was rarely unemotional. I would be anxious, rueful, beleaguered, furious, frustrated, sad. There were moments, too, of warmth, gratitude, laughter, joy, relief, even love. I was never, ever bored—the experience that had driven me from that long-ago suburban practice. I was always interested in the patient before me. Their problems engaged me, even when I'd heard them a million times before, even when I thought they were phony or pedestrian or overblown. The lies could be more interesting than the truths. I would enter the exam room and everything else would fall away, except for the issues at hand. My focus would be absolute. This capacity I had surprises even me. It came without effort. Of all my foibles as a clinician, the failure to attend to the patient and her story was not one of them.

Then, without warning, here I was with this man, shrinking away from his words, thinking to myself, *I don't want to hear this. I don't care about your problem. It was sobering.*

I'd entered my twenty-eighth year in practice, all but three of them spent working with marginalized populations. Two years earlier I had abandoned my medical directorship of two decades and returned to medicine full time.

My day began around 7:30 and ended between 5:30 and 6:00. The pace was grueling. No breaks, only jokes about holding it, because there was scarcely time to pee. My administrative work life, in contrast, had seemed leisurely, with an extravagance of time to reflect on problems and projects. In the clinic, I took no breaks. I brought my lunch and ate while I worked. Coffee and foodstuff stained the desk. I wore slacks, loose sweaters or jackets, and sensible shoes. I drew back my hair with combs to make sure it would never fall into my eyes and would hold up all day in a professionally acceptable fashion without further fussing. I only had time to comb it once, in the morning. What the day demanded felt faintly athletic.

The patients were generally gone by 4:30, the staff by 5:00. In the after-hours still of the clinic I would review labs and reports, formulate plans, document them in the charts. Not infrequently I would puzzle over an unexpectedly abnormal test. Did it signify something important? Should I repeat it? Were there additional exams I should order? Not every irregularity merited pursuit. A diagnostic chase after a marginal abnormality could be just as easily fruitless, wasteful, even harmful, as helpful. Among my patients, abnormal tests were legion. I couldn't possibly work up all of them. I would break the bank and end up with nothing to show for it. It was a judgment call. Nothing was for certain. And at 5:45, after ten unrelieved hours of cognitive labor, I would be stumped. I would close the record and leave it. The next morning I would open it up again and I would see immediately what my plan should be.

It was the evening of my career and there would be no morning to follow. No fresh start. I was tired and more demoralized and cynical than I cared to admit. A suspicion had plagued me all the years of my practice that I was not cut out for this work, that I did not have the required psychological fortitude, that becoming a doctor was the biggest mistake of my life. That I had only managed all these years because my exposure was part time. This unhappy thought visited me more frequently during these waning years of my practice.

Over the course of my time in medicine our understanding of pathology had advanced astronomically; the number of drugs and diagnostics had increased likewise. So much more was crammed into the same twenty minutes. The clinical project was vastly more complicated; it was impossible to keep up. Regular conferences, trainings, and the reading of journals were not enough. In primary care nothing fenced in the body of material the doctor was supposed to master. It was boundless. No wonder that more than three-quarters of doctors were choosing more focused, as well as more lucrative, careers in the specialties.[13]

Over the years I had watched a number of my primary care colleagues bail out. It felt like it was time to follow. My daily objective had slipped from helping my patient achieve a greater sense of well-being to conducting a safe clinical encounter, to making no mistakes. Every day felt like a set-up for failure, and the stakes were high. And now, I was losing interest as well. A year later, I retired.

❦

The clinic threw a party for me and sent invitations to my patients, at least those with addresses. Word got around and lots of patients came. We staged the party in the waiting room of our recently remodeled clinic.

A chief impetus for the remodel was to accommodate a new kind of service delivery, the patient-centered, primary care home model. Each patient was assigned to a team, which consisted of two primary care providers and a psych NP, nurses, medical assistants, a social worker, and a clerk. Continuity and quality of care were significantly improved. Patients loved it and the staff grew to love it as well. It made so much sense. It embodied what I miss most about my practice: collaborating with like-minded individuals on a meaningful project.

One consequence of the remodel was loss of the only windows in reception, which made the ceiling appear lower and the space more cave-like. Still the room was less institutional, more colorful, and the atmosphere more soothing. It no longer looked like a place where you'd expect to see broken chairs, someone passed out in the corner, and cockroaches scurrying along the walls. Between reception and the back office, locked doors were installed, a security precaution. What a far cry from our Burnside Clinic. Funding ran out before the remodel was finished, so most of the exam rooms did not get the snazzy new floors installed in the clinic below us.

Staff did not get much time to enjoy the new space. Westside Health Center closed less than two years after I retired, and staff were relocated to a clinic outside the downtown area. Our longstanding partner, Central City Concern, agreed to take on our patients. CCC had taken over management of Old Town Clinic in 2001 from its solo practitioner and built an array of cutting-edge clinical services for the homeless and other impoverished residents of downtown. They are very good at what they do.

Three of my physician colleagues at Westside retired shortly before or after I did. Between us, we had close to one hundred years of experience working with underserved populations. Many factors led to the demise of the clinic, but chief among them was the inability to recruit new docs. Interest in a primary care career among newly minted physicians fell to historic lows during the first decade of the millennium,[14] at the same time the demand for primary care was rising. Every system in town was recruiting for primary care docs. Salary offerings were climbing. The Health Department couldn't compete. And perhaps practicing among the poor did not offer the same attraction for a new generation of doctors as it did for those of us who came of age in the sixties.

❧

I have photos from the party. I pull them up on my computer for the first time since I left the clinic. This writing has rendered me morose. The photos are a good antidote.

Here I am, arm in arm with a stocky guy who, after years of congeniality, had one day blown up at me in the most paranoid and inexplicable fashion. Two weeks later, it was as if nothing had ever happened. He no longer lives.

In this photo, I'm draped over the shoulders of a fellow in a wheelchair. By the time he came to me, he could no longer walk, because in prison a pressure on his spinal cord had been ignored until the damage was irreparable.

The lady with the long black hair, who used to wear all red clothing, makeup, and nail polish, stands with her arms around me. Once she achieved some psychiatric stability, she'd gained weight and ceased her monochromatic approach to wardrobe. I'd known her for more than twenty years. I was the only mom she'd ever had, she'd once told me.

There's a shot of me with an asthmatic woman. When she managed to quit smoking after years of trying, my nurse, Karen Hogue, who'd invested nothing short of her own soul into this patient, brought in cupcakes and threw a small celebration for the patient and her mother.

And seated with his grin and his guitar is yet another man, African-American, who was said to be both intellectually impaired and schizophrenic. The day we'd met, he'd been so terrified of me, he wouldn't let me touch the painful callous he'd brought in to show his new doctor. In the photo, he's treating me to a sweet serenade.

❧

When I knew I would be leaving, something fell loose inside. That professional distance I'd cultivated, by which I mean keeping my personal life out of the exam room, ceased to matter so much. To those who expressed interest, I spoke about my family, my husband and my boy (no longer a boy), and my interests outside of medicine. I began to hug patients more and kiss their drawn or pudgy or sallow cheeks. I held more hands. Lots of them I called sweetie.

I was, however, never promiscuous with my affections. Many, maybe most of the patients, neither desired nor could tolerate this kind of closeness. A minority would even misinterpret it, abuse it, take advantage. These patients were usually easy to spot. The ones, for example, who called me by my first name without an invitation. Lots of my patients used my given name, whoever was comfortable with the informality, whoever did not need to hold intact in her mind a professional image of me. But an occasional person, whose manner revealed a certain sense of entitlement, lack of respect, even insolence, took the liberty as a way of asserting himself against me. Or as a way to manufacture a chumminess he calculated would seduce me into giving him whatever he wanted. I realize in writing this I've changed gender pronouns. Because these guys were all guys. I would never hug such a patient or bestow on him an endearment.

But for others, especially the ones I'd cared for over a span of years, this miniscule sharing of the not-doctor parts of me and the demonstrations of affection added a satisfying depth to the relationship. It was not how I was taught to behave with patients, and I wished that I had fallen to it much earlier.

❧

The ways that I kept my home life out of the clinic never worked so well in reverse. I brought the clinic home, or it came home of its own accord. For example, as a fifteen-year-old, Alex happened to field one call from a patient bent on harassing me. He was proud of his restrained and firm performance. My husband Norm, who is wise in all sorts of ways, often provided a sounding board for me to work out a difficult problem, though not those of a precisely clinical nature, as he is not a medical doctor himself.

The smallest intrusions were the worst, less disruptive but more grinding. As Alex pointed out already as a kid, in his generous and understated way, at the end of a clinic day I was, all too often, irritable. All I wanted to do was eat and collapse. My work was intensely social, and I was not. The care of patients is a great set-up for an introvert, the encounters structured and scripted. I could be with people in meaningful ways without having to worry about any kind of social improvisation, for which I had no aptitude. But the time in clinic emptied me out. I would straggle home emotionally depleted, with little space left in heart or mind to accommodate either my husband or my son, though I doubt they would state it so baldly. Or maybe only my husband would. Kids are more forgiving.

If Norm was happy that I had retired, I was deliriously so. I let my DEA certification, my board certification, and finally my license lapse. The journal subscriptions tapered off. To the many who inquired if I missed it, I replied, "Nope, not for a second." I soon lost count of the number who remarked: "You look so much more relaxed and happy."

§

In this photo you can't see that half of the woman's left leg is missing, lost to an infection from shooting up. She's clean and sober and grateful and has taken me into her arms. A few years later I will learn of her death from an overdose.

This smiley fellow once made me a card of a photo he'd taken, which captured the spire of the First Presbyterian Church and the imposing edifice of the Elks Temple, backed by a rainbow. Enough symbols, he'd joked, of earthly and celestial power for one image. He's gone, too, succumbed to the ravages of a rare and chronic disorder.

Barry Mattern is there. He tries not to weep and fails.

The Native American woman who'd lived on the street as long as I had known her, with terrible liver disease and equally terrible judgment about the company she keeps, has glommed on to me the way a child does, every part of her pressed into me. She has an expression on her round face as she hugs me that I can only describe as beatific.

Another patient, a lapsed man of the cloth, claims a space at my side for the camera. Later, the ex-journalist, whom I always thought might be a good companion for the ex-minister, poses with me, as well. Both of them are smart and thoughtful. But I don't introduce them.

There are more. In every single photo my smile is immense. In every one I'm jammed up against a patient, cheek to cheek, my arms wrapped around them or theirs around me.

NOTES TO THE TEXT

1   Darrel A. Regier, MD, MPH et al., "Comorbidity of Mental Disorders with Alcohol and Other Drug Abuse: Results from the Epidemiologic Catchment Area (ECA) Study," *Journal of the American Medical Association* 264, no. 19 (November 21, 1990): 2511–2518.

2   Jay C. Fournier et al., "Antidepressant Drug Effects and Depression Severity: A Patient-Level Meta-analysis," *Journal of the American Medical Association* 303, no. 1 (January 6, 2010): 47–53.

3   MH Teicher et al., "Emergence of Intense Suicidal Preoccupation during Fluoxetine Treatment," *American Journal of Psychiatry* 147, no. 2 (February 1990): 207–210.

4   Padmini Varadarajan, MD et al., "Clinical Profile and Natural History of 453 Nonsurgically Managed Patients with Severe Aortic Stenosis," *Annals of Thoracic Surgery* 82 (July 2006): 2111–2115.

5   Jerome Groopman, *How Doctors Think* (New York: Houghton Mifflin, 2007).

6   Kimberly S. H. Yarnall, et al., "Primary Care: Is There Enough Time for Prevention?" *American Journal of Public Health* 93, no. 4 (April 2003): 635–641.

7   S. Brown et al., "Twenty-five Year Mortality of a Community Cohort with Schizophrenia," *British Journal of Psychiatry* 196 (February 2010): 116–121; Tim J R Lambert and John W. Newcomer, "Are the Cardiometabolic Complications of Schizophre-

nia Still Neglected? Barriers to Care," *Medical Journal of Australia* 190, no. 4 (February 16, 2009); Sukanta Saha, MSc, MCN et al., "A Systematic Review of Mortality in Schizophrenia: Is the Differential Mortality Gap Worsening Over Time?" *Archives of General Psychiatry* 64, no. 10 (October 2007): 1123–1131.

8   Even Myrbakk and Stephen Von Tetzchner, "Psychiatric Disorders and Behavior Problems in People with Intellectual Disability," *Research in Developmental Disabilities* 29 (2008): 316–332.

9   FC Blow et al., "Ethnicity and Diagnostic Patterns in Veterans with Psychoses," *Social Psychiatry & Psychiatric Epidemiology* 39, no. 10 (2004): 841–851; Javier Escobar, "Diagnostic Bias: Racial and Cultural Issues," *Psychiatric Services* (ps.psychiatryonline.org) 63, no. 9 (September 2012): 847.

10   Jonathan M. Metzl, *The Protest Psychosis: How Schizophrenia Became a Black Disease* (Boston: Beacon Press, 2011).

11   Myrbakk, "Psychiatric Disorders," 316–332 (see note 8).

12   Brent Walth, "Moving the Needle: A New Law Expanding the Use of an Anti-overdose Drug is Cutting the Number of Heroin Deaths," *Willamette Week* (April 15, 2014).

13   Phillips, Robert L. Jr, MD, MSPH et al., "Specialty and Geographic Distribution of the Physician Workforce: What Influences Medical Student and Resident Choices?", (Washington, DC, The Robert Graham Center: Policy Studies in Family Medicine and Primary Care, 2009).

14   Ibid.